The Natural Pregnancy Book

# THE
# Natural Pregnancy Book

THIRD EDITION

Your Complete Guide to a Safe,
Organic Pregnancy and Childbirth
with Herbs, Nutrition, and
Other Holistic Choices

Aviva Jill Romm

Foreword by Ina May Gaskin

TEN SPEED PRESS
Berkeley

The information contained in this book is based on the experience and research of the author. It is not intended as a substitute for consulting with your physician or other health care provider. Any attempt to diagnose and treat an illness should be done under the direction of a health care professional. The publisher does not advocate the use of any particular health care protocol, but believes that the information in this book should be available to the public. The publisher and author are not responsible for any adverse effects or consequences resulting from the use of any of the suggestions, preparations, or procedures discussed in this book. Should the reader have any questions concerning the appropriateness of any procedure or preparation mentioned, the author and publisher strongly suggest consulting a professional health care advisor.

Copyright © 1997, 2003, 2014 by Aviva Jill Romm
Illustrations © 1997, 2003 by Marna Groves
All rights reserved.

Published in the United States by Ten Speed Press, an imprint of the Crown Publishing Group, a division of Random House LLC, a Penguin Random House Company, New York.
www.crownpublishing.com
www.tenspeed.com

Ten Speed Press and the Ten Speed Press colophon are registered trademarks of Random House LLC.

Previous editions published in 1997 by Crossing Press, Freedom, California, and in 2003 by Celestial Arts, Berkeley, California.

Library of Congress Cataloging-in-Publication Data
Romm, Aviva Jill.
The natural pregnancy book : your complete guide to a safe, organic pregnancy and childbirth with herbs, nutrition, and other holistic choices / Aviva Jill Romm ; foreword by Ina May Gaskin.
— Third edition.
     pages cm
1. Pregnancy—Popular works. 2. Holistic medicine—Popular works. 3. Alternative medicine—Popular works. I. Title.
 RG525.R675 2014
 618.2—dc23

2014008356

Trade Paperback ISBN: 978-1-60774-448-1
eBook ISBN: 978-1-60774-449-8

Printed in the United States of America

Design by Chloe Rawlins

10 9 8 7 6 5 4 3 2 1

Third Edition

*This book is dedicated to all of the women who have,*
*over the centuries, kept women's wisdom alive—*
*it is because of their courage that I am here today; to my husband,*
*Tracy Romm, and to our children, Iyah, Yemima, Forest, and Naomi;*
*to my sister-in-law, Felicity Romm, and her children,*
*Serenity, Caleb, and Keziah Romm, for their incredible strength;*
*and finally, to the spirit of my brother-in-law, Chip Romm.*

# Contents

# Acknowledgments

⟫⟫⟫⟪⟪⟪

*This book could not have been written* without the unfailing support of my mate, Tracy Romm. Tracy is truly a midwife's advocate, a man who understands what it means for me to leave home in the middle of the night to wipe a woman's brow, say a few encouraging words, and be honored to greet a new member of our human family—while he scrambles to juggle his own work schedule to accommodate my work. He also knows what it takes to "midwife" a book—and he has been my unfailing assistant in the process. He has joyfully played with, fed, read to, and nurtured our four children during the numerous hours it took to write this book— and in the intervening years since the first edition was published. And he has encouraged me to keep writing because he cares so much about those who might benefit—the next generations, as well as our own.

I am overjoyed by and thankful for the presence of my four children—my son, Iyah Khalil, my stalwart supporter and ardent encourager; and my three daughters, Yemima Shanti, who at six said, "Mom, you're an awesome woman!" and at fourteen says, "Mom, you get more beautiful every day," and my Forest Grace and Naomi Shoshannah, who played the most magical games by my side as I typed away on these keys when they were babies, and who now, during these revisions, have grown into strong and competent young people. These four people have shared me generously with the world, and I am honored to be their mom.

I would like to thank all of the midwives, herbalists, and healers who have been my teachers, friends, and inspiration—too numerous to mention, but you know who you are! A special place in my heart is reserved for Sarahn Henderson, my soul sister, midwife, and teacher; Lizzie McDaniels-Feigenbaum, Lisa Olko, and Kim Land, who shared the journeys of motherhood and midwifery with me in important ways. I also want to offer a special word of honor to Ina May Gaskin for being my original inspiration—it was her book *Spiritual Midwifery,* which found its way to me when I was fifteen, that really opened my eyes to being a midwife—and to the late Jeannine Parvati Baker for welcoming me into the herbal and midwifery sisterhood. Also, thanks to my friends in the herbal world for their support and encouragement of my work in my fledgling years: Michael Tierra, Susun Weed, and Rosemary Gladstar.

Thanks to Elaine Gill and the staff at The Crossing Press for originally recognizing that this book needed to be published and for having full faith in me, and to the folks at Celestial Arts for making my dreams come true by bringing this book into the fold. Also, thanks go to Dr. Richard Clofine for carefully reviewing the manuscript and having the guts to support it as an obstetrician. And thank you Emily Timberlake and Ten Speed Press, for believing in keeping this book alive so new generations can benefit from its old and new wisdom.

Finally, I am eternally grateful to the families that have welcomed me into the sacred space of their pregnancies, and who have called me, with joy, their midwife.

# Foreword by Ina May Gaskin

꘎꘎꘎꘎꘍꘍꘍

*When I was pregnant* for the first time back in 1965, I naively supposed there must be a book that would answer the questions that continuously bubbled up in my mind. How was I to stay within the twelve- to fifteen-pound weight gain allowed by my obstetrician and not be constantly hungry? Why was this weight limit necessary? What should I expect when I went into labor? How was I to learn how to take care of a baby? How did maternal instincts develop? (I thought I was sadly lacking in this department because I hadn't played with baby dolls as a child.) I searched both the university and public libraries in my town for the book I wanted but came up with nothing.

My obstetrician was of little or no help in answering my questions because he always seemed to be in a hurry—even though I never saw anyone else in his waiting room. In fact, for all I knew, I was the only pregnant woman in that small midwestern town where I was attending graduate school. Not once during this pregnancy did I talk to anyone (besides my obstetrician) who was either pregnant or claimed to know anything about pregnancy. Obtaining a midwife was totally out of the question—in fact, doing that never once occurred to me, because I was unaware there was any such being in all of the United States.

It was at my last prenatal visit before going into labor that my obstetrician informed me that since this was my first baby, I would be having a forceps delivery. When I protested, he interrupted to tell me that a natural birth of a first-time mother was likely to result in a brain-damaged baby. Unconvinced, I decided the best strategy for avoiding a forceps delivery—I knew from reading historical novels that forceps could cause brain damage—was to be the quietest woman ever to have a baby in that hospital.

It didn't work. My baby was pulled out by forceps, despite how silently I had labored. She wasn't brain damaged, but she and I were both negatively affected for many years by the psychological separation that stemmed from our physical separation for nearly twenty-four hours after her birth, and I felt that her birth had been something that had happened to me instead of something that I had done.

Young mothers these days do not have to worry about unnecessary forceps deliveries because this fashion in obstetrics, once so widely and uncritically accepted in our country, is now as extinct as the pterodactyl. There are now far more books available on pregnancy and childbirth than most women have time to read or money to buy, and childbirth classes are available to probably the majority of women in the United States. Husbands, partners, family members, and even friends are allowed in the labor and delivery rooms of most hospitals, and it is a common, if mistaken, perception that childbirth is now handled in the best way possible.

The reality is far less reassuring. For one thing, not all of the books are that helpful. Many contain misleading information or even misinformation. As for interventions in the process of pregnancy, labor, and birth, it is now possible— even likely—for American women to have unnecessary ultrasonography during pregnancy, unnecessary inductions, unnecessary intravenous feedings, unnecessary electronic fetal monitoring, and unnecessary anesthesia during labor. Needless cesarean sections reached epidemic proportions in the United States during the 1970s and have remained at historically high levels ever since, despite the strenuous efforts of consumer organizations such as the International Cesarean Awareness Network (ICAN) to lower them and despite the repeated recommendations by the obstetricians' own professional organization, the American College of Obstetricians and Gynecologists (ACOG).

Because, after fifty years of concerted efforts to revive the profession of midwifery in the United States, there are still only a few thousand midwives available to attend the four million births that happen annually, not every woman is going to be able to find a midwife to provide her prenatal care and to attend her birth.

Regardless of whether you have a midwife or are one of the women who cannot obtain midwifery care, Aviva's book is going to be a comfort to you. She understands as a mother and as a midwife what you are going through, and she has an uncommon gift of writing down her knowledge in a way that is accessible and graceful. Read it and be nurtured.

# Preface

*This book was conceived* nearly thirty years ago in the kitchen of a dear friend's home. At that time, she and I, both midwives and each the mother of a young child, were beginning a lifetime journey of uncovering and rediscovering a great wealth of information about childbearing and child raising. We were gleaning information from a variety of sources: anthropological research, medical and lay texts, our work as mothers and midwives, the experiences of other midwives and mothers, and, most significantly, what we were learning from our intuition, from each other as women friends, from our partnerships with our mates, and from our babies. We had found that pregnancy did not have to be ten (lunar) months of drudgery, discomfort, and exhaustion. We were finding that pregnancy and motherhood could be highly creative times, filled with confidence, perceptiveness, awe, and appreciation for the beauty of our changing physical shape, and the extension of this in the form of our growing children.

Standing in the doorway of that kitchen on an early spring day, a moment ripe for beginnings, I found an inspiration and made the commitment to carry this inspiration inside me, to gestate and nurture my discoveries until, like a baby after a full-term pregnancy, a book would be ready to emerge, to be born—a book to share the joy and strength I was gaining from my experiences. That so many women see pregnancy as a burden to be endured, a time fraught with insecurity and doubt, seemed a great loss. Aware of the transformative potential of the written word, I became determined to contribute a positive, supportive narrative about pregnancy by a woman and mother, for women and mothers everywhere.

I now have four children, all of whom have grown and flourished in their own unique and significant ways. I've had healthy pregnancies, strong labors, and beautiful births. I've nursed my babies and deeply enjoyed each of our children through every stage of childhood, adolescence, and unfolding adulthood. Each pregnancy has reaffirmed my conviction that natural health care is the bedrock of continuing wellness for myself and my family, and watching my children develop into strong, healthy beings has only strengthened that principle. In addition to my own pregnancies, I have had the honor to know and assist many women and families on the mostly joyous, sometimes tumultuous, and occasionally painful path of pregnancy. I experienced life come full circle this past January when I served as the midwife for the birth of my first grandchild. The joy I felt as I witnessed and supported my baby as he experienced the birth of his baby was transcendent, otherworldly, a moment that far exceeded any fantasy I could have dreamed up.

As women have become increasingly aware of the options of natural birth and home birth, and of the potential value of natural therapies as safe alternatives to some of the conventional medical treatments of common pregnancy complaints, I have watched with pride and elation as this book has found renewed purpose. Today it speaks to more than a piqued group of concerned alternative thinkers; it speaks to a diverse population of women and mothers who are curious about taking control of their health, their bodies, and their pregnancies. The face of wellness has changed since this book was first published, and there is now welcomed emphasis on natural treatments, herbal medicine, and integrative support. It is a pleasure to share this book—one of the original voices in the world of natural health for mommas—with you. The wisdom and information within it stands the test of time.

PART I

# Your Pregnancy

# CHAPTER 1

# The Basics

>>><<<

*The Natural Pregnancy Book* is written for you, regardless of how extensively you want to use natural remedies. Whether you simply wish to have a relaxed and healthy pregnancy and be knowledgeable about the process or you actually want to dive deeper into the worlds of nutrition and herbs, you can gain a great deal from this book with its sections on nutrition, movement, and relaxation, as well as common natural remedies for common pregnancy concerns. If you aren't pregnant yet, but would like to be, you can use this book as part of you preparation for entering pregnancy in optimal health.

Grandmothers, aunts, sisters, friends, and partners of pregnant women can read this book to re-create the support systems that women have relied upon for generations, both during pregnancy and after the baby is born. This book will enable these people to be a positive and nourishing influence for the pregnant woman.

Women who are interested in what is known in our country as "alternative healing," "holistic medicine," "complementary medicine," or "natural health" will find this book one they turn to again and again for practical methods of relieving common pregnancy discomforts and promoting optimal health in pregnancy.

This book is addressed to you as the pregnant momma, because pregnancy, although it offers a transformational experience for our partners (if they're in the picture), is a woman's experience, one that a woman can, and I believe should, claim as her own. With this sense of ownership of your body and pregnancy, I hope will come a sense of confidence to make choices and be the creative agent of your prenatal care.

Pregnancy is a time rich in possibility for relationship building between the parents and baby, even while the baby is still gestating. Hopefully, involved partners will read much of this book too. Chapter 13 is written primarily for fathers but should also be read as inclusive to all partners—I am so happy that nontraditional relationships aren't as nontraditional as when this book was first written!

## A Brief History of Birthing Practices in the United States

Approximately four million women in the United States give birth every year. The majority continue to choose physicians as their care providers—usually obstetricians, sometimes family doctors. Until recently only about 4 percent (about 160,000 women) received care from midwives. In 2009, there was a spike up to 8 percent—an all-time high. Less than 2 percent of women choose home births—though the popularity of this option is also growing. Yet it is well established that midwives provide safer, less interventional, more personalized, and more cost-effective care than other providers.

Prior to the twentieth century, most women used midwives and gave birth at home; what happened in women's choice of care provider? Early in the twentieth century, the midwife's role was usurped by medical doctors with final control assumed by obstetricians. Doctors and hospitals began to be perceived as safer and more desirable than midwives and home births. In fact, in those days there was greater danger of women dying in childbirth in hospitals due to sepsis from uterine infections spread by physicians who failed to wash their hands between patients.

With the shift toward hospitals and obstetricians, women's role became less active in giving birth to their babies. Technology encouraged passivity. Standard obstetric language described birth as women being "delivered"—and it was true—women were unable to participate in the process with their legs in stirrups high in the air, wrist straps to hold them immobile, and *twilight sleep* (partial loss of consciousness via anesthetics) to keep them mostly unconscious. This shift also led to excessive use of forceps deliveries and an eventual increase in cesarean sections.

In the late 1960s, with the help of the Women's Rights Movement, women began to take back birth. Encouraged by various new childbirth methods promoted by Frederick Leboyer, Grantly Dick-Read, and the Lamaze movement, there was a renewed emphasis on a more natural approach to birth. Women began to ask their partners to participate in their pregnancies and births, and it became commonplace for men to do so. Nevertheless, with all these advances, women were still cast in stereotypical compliant roles.

In the 1970s and 1980s, technology was increasingly emphasized in obstetrical care. Due to legal and financial considerations on the part of many doctors, hospitals, medical supply houses, and insurance companies, prenatal and intrapartum testing became requisite for all pregnant women rather than optional and for those at higher risk. Women as a whole did not question this growing number of interventions or their consequences. At that time, there was no evidence of a movement to limit the growing over-medicalization of childbirth, with the exception of a very small number of "back to the landers" scattered throughout the United States, who were having their babies at home in cabins, teepees, and school buses (a famous example being the women at The Farm, in rural Tennessee).

Well into the 1980s, most women were still not informed about pregnancy and birth, and obstetrics all but absolved us of our responsibility. We were still patronized, frequently drugged, strapped down for birth—but now not literally to the table but to external fetal monitors—and subject to isolating and inconsiderate treatment. Babies were still held upside down directly after birth, slapped, and whisked away from their mothers. Few women breastfed their babies.

*The open heart, freed from fear, experiences the world, in all its mystery and brilliance. All of us need to practice awe-robics, like Lily Tomlin's character, Trudy.*

—DIANE MARIECHILD

Despite some gains in equal rights in the workplace and home, women are still not the decision makers in their pregnancies and birthing experiences. Women had political control over childbearing when it was a private, women's experience, but they lost control of that and let the medical establishment become the authority. It has been only recently, nearly twenty years after the original publication of this book, that women have begun to question contemporary birthing practices. Movies such as *Business of Baby* have shed light on the now unacceptably high cesarean section rate, which is greater than 33 percent nationwide.

Never before have pregnant women been expected to subject themselves to the level of prenatal testing, screening, and diagnosis that they are now. Because of our tendency to believe unquestioningly in medical experts, we allow ourselves and our babies to undergo practices that we are told are safe but medical literature often cites as harmful. This book offers suggestions for a different model of care but also documents medical techniques that women might choose or need. This book is a compilation of the best that the tradition of midwifery has to offer in noninvasive methods for promoting and maintaining pregnancy wellness. It is a woman-to-woman guide to pregnancy care.

I believe that pregnancy is a natural process of which our bodies are perfectly capable and that it has the potential for being a process of growth and initiation into a value system that respects and honors women's creative power, rather than how this process is currently perceived—as a time when we give up our power to medical authorities who infantilize us.

This book is therefore woman centered and feminist. I firmly believe that women are the best authorities on our own bodies. Also, childbearing is a women's rights issue when it is happening in the context of a medical system that can deny our freedom to choose where, how, and with whom we want to birth our babies, and in a system where a woman could be court ordered to make decisions against her actual will.

This book invites women to claim our bodies' processes as a part of our strength, not of our weakness, and to work together for the empowerment of women. I believe that reclaiming pregnancy should be part of our collective effort for broad-reaching social change in all aspects of women's health care.

While this book offers many alternatives to conventional medical care, it is not antimedical, antihospital, or anti-obstetrician. As a midwife, I have seen truly necessary medical interventions and have been thankful for their skillful employment; have met dedicated and caring physicians, nurses, and nurse-midwives; and have seen great improvements in hospitals. What I take issue with is the inappropriate use of technology and the attitude that pregnancy is an illness.

This book strives to help you reframe your thinking so you can regain your natural authority. Through the development of our own voice and story, trust in our ability to understand common medical rationale and practices, and confidence in our capability for competent decision making, we can feel more fully empowered to transform the cultural stereotypes that undermine the potential for positive growth and transformation inherent in the pregnancy experience.

The *Natural Pregnancy Book* is devoted not only to helping women gain trust and respect for their birthing abilities, but also to teaching that what we do in pregnancy matters for our children's long-term physical, psychological, and social health. When I first wrote this book, my ideas about avoiding unnecessary environmental exposures (including to many chemicals, medications, and even prolonged stress) were radical ideas—now it is well known that by the time of birth, babies are already inundated with exposures that can lead to later development of asthma, diabetes, autism, and cancer! This book was an early clarion call—my views on the need for a natural pregnancy to protect our kids have become even stronger and are backed by substantial scientific evidence.

It is my sincerest hope that this book will inspire you to listen to and respect your body and to find the empowerment that will allow you to take a stand for the type of pregnancy and birth experience you and your baby deserve. May this be a gift that we pass on to our daughters and sons, that they too may respect themselves, and each other.

## What I Mean by Natural

The term *natural childbirth* has been reduced by the obstetrics community to mean any birth that occurs vaginally (as opposed to a cesarean section), regardless of whether there have been interventions or the use of medications. While it is a disservice to a woman to feel guilty if she ultimately decides to have an epidural, for example, to call such a birth "natural" trivializes the common use of drugs and interventions during both pregnancy and birth and dilutes the likelihood of women recognizing that it is possible and empowering to experience a pregnancy and birth that is free of unnecessary intrusions or interventions. When I use the word *natural*, I am referring to untampered-with and unhindered biological processes, techniques that support such healthy biological functioning, and substances that are primarily derived from unrefined sources.

A natural approach to pregnancy necessitates that you respect the forces of your body—those that cause conception to occur and that also cause your baby to grow in your womb—and that you try to work in harmony with those forces by bringing elements from the natural world (for example, foods in their natural state and herbs) into your pregnancy experience.

## Alternative Childbirth and the Resurgence of Midwifery

In the mid-1970s, a small but determined number of women began to question the type of treatment they were receiving from the medical profession in their pregnancy and birth experiences. Coincident with the rise of the women's self-help movement and the so-called back-to-the-land movement, women began to turn to a more traditional and natural approach to pregnancy and birth, relying more on trust in natural cycles for reassurance of their wellness than on medical advice and testing. A resurgence in midwifery care, home birth, and the use of practical self-care began. Some of the earliest pioneers of this movement include

Ina May Gaskin, Sheila Kitzinger, Jeannine Parvati Baker, Elizabeth Davis, Raven Lang, Nan Koehler, Suzanne Arms, and Rahima Baldwin, as well as the midwives who founded the Childbirth Providers of African Descent—Shafia Monroe, Sondra Abdullah Zaimah, Ayanna Ade, and Rashida Mujtabah—and countless other women whose persistent and courageous efforts have kept natural birth options open for all of us.

With the growth of this alternative childbirth movement, midwives and mothers had available to them both the best natural traditions and the best advanced obstetrical knowledge on which to draw. In fact, many midwives were women who wanted to provide other women with the type of care that they wished they had received during pregnancy. Women began to teach childbirth education classes, and some of them, such as sociologist and anthropologist Sheila Kitzinger and midwife and educator Rahima Baldwin, founded international organizations to inform and empower pregnant women. A handful of supportive physicians also provided assistance for those desiring a more natural approach to pregnancy and birth.

By the 1980s, the alternative birth movement had gained momentum, and though less than 1 percent of all women chose home births, midwifery was no longer a thing of the past. With the resurgence of midwifery came a resurgence of the prejudice against women healers and the attendant persecution of midwives. In many areas of the United States, traditional midwives have been arrested, harassed, and faced with restraint-of-trade charges, and have endured emotional and economic hardships as a result of court cases and legal fees. Of course, the families of these practitioners have suffered greatly as well. Even certified nurse-midwives, fully trained and sanctioned by the medical establishment, are typically required to practice under the auspices of an obstetrician. Individual obstetricians as well as the regulating organization of nurse-midwives determine just how much autonomy a nurse-midwife is allowed.

In 1982, in an effort to consolidate knowledge and create internal midwifery standards as well as to provide a consistent forum for education, midwives across the United States formed the Midwives Alliance of North America, an organization that now has an international membership and is working to foster public acceptance and recognition of independent midwifery, not only as a respected profession but also as an option available to a greater spectrum of women. This is in keeping with the belief that midwifery is political and is social work that extends beyond small circles of "back-to-nature" women who choose to have babies at home. Midwives are committed to the care of pregnant women and are working to create a political environment in which all women have the option of receiving the kind of care and support midwives offer—professional care that is nurturing and designed to meet the needs of individual women.

The alternative childbirth movement has had a significant impact on women's experiences of childbirth, even for those choosing to give birth conventionally and in the hospital. The development of birth plans; prevalence of birthing rooms; presence of fathers, friends, and children at births; availability of birthing balls and birthing tubs; reduced episiotomy rates; increased breastfeeding; and more are all testaments to the efforts of the alternative childbirth movement. The growing popularity of organic eating during pregnancy, exercise and yoga for prenatal relaxation and toning, and attention to holistic and spiritual health, including the use of herbs, massage, and meditation, also reflect the influence of the alternative birth movement on mainstream pregnancy and birthing practices.

## Looking to the Future

Even though there has been a lot of positive change in how we approach pregnancy and birth, this is just a veneer over the surface of increasing medicalization. Despite birthing rooms, more midwives, better breastfeeding rates, and the appearance of natural options, the cesarean section rate in the United States is one of the highest in the world. We also have one of the highest obstetric intervention rates in the world, and we rank unfavorably in neonatal outcomes.

The rates of interventions have been escalating. The reality is, due to our fierce desires to protect our babies at all costs, we still hand over our responsibility to the medical profession starting at the first prenatal visit and continuing through the birth and beyond into pediatric care. At a time when a woman should be developing into a confident parent, the medical profession in general deals a severe blow to that developing confidence by making her dependent upon its experts for direction. If we have not already been indoctrinated into the medical system by the time we reach pregnancy, then surely we will be—unless we choose differently.

*Midwives are committed to the care of pregnant women and are working to create a political environment in which all women have the option of receiving the kind of care and support midwives offer—professional care that is nurturing, designed to meet the needs of individual women.* ⫸

I am not suggesting that we abandon all medical care during pregnancy (though for many women, care can be obtained entirely through midwives!). I do question the routine use of unnecessary and invasive practices. Further, women who choose to forgo such prenatal testing should not be penalized emotionally—or legally.

I propose that we consider what it would be like to regain confidence in ourselves, beginning with the experiences that our bodies present to us through our reproductive cycles, if not before. Regaining confidence in our bodies, it seems to me, is the most challenging aspect in overcoming what we have lost in our complex history of childbearing.

It is within our grasp as women and mothers to determine what pregnancy and prenatal care will be in the twenty-first century. Will we become convinced that technological intervention is a wiser choice than heeding our bodies' natural processes? Or will we welcome these processes and come to view our bodies—indeed, ourselves—with respect for our strengths, power, and beauty?

# CHAPTER 2

# Becoming Body Centered

>>>⟨⟨⟨

*We live in a culture* where most of us relate to our bodies not by how we feel but by how we think we look. We judge ourselves against the images we see around us, even airbrushed images of pregnant celebrities on fashion magazine covers! Basing our feelings about our bodies on our appearance leads enormous numbers of women into dangerous patterns. Dieting—rather than nutrition—is a major focus for many women. Studies report that in the 1980s and 1990s there was an explosion of eating disorders. An estimated eight million American women are reported as anorexic, bulimic, or compulsive dieters.

Commercials and advertisements offer an array of convenient products that will make our bodies cleaner and more pleasant smelling. What are the effects on our psyches of such an implied contempt for the female body and the view of its functions as fundamentally dirty? Do we have to "sanitize" our bodies to make them conform to external standards? Or can we learn to love our bodies and listen to them?

In *Women's Bodies, Women's Wisdom*, Dr. Christiane Northrup, an obstetrician and gynecologist and a specialist in holistic health for women, writes, "The state of a woman's health is indeed completely tied up with the culture in which she lives and her position in it, as well as in the way she lives her life as an individual. We cannot hope to reclaim our bodily wisdom and inherent ability to create health without first understanding the influence of our society on how we think and care for our bodies." How we think about and care for our bodies is the basis for how we feel during pregnancy. Therefore, it is important to look at some of the underlying beliefs and attitudes that women in our culture are exposed to and too often internalize. By understanding and redefining your relationship with your body, you will be improving the likelihood that you can experience pregnancy as a positive and magical process.

Not only does popular media cause us to distrust our bodies' natural processes, but the medical profession, into whose hands most of us were literally born, has conditioned us to rely on its experts for answers to our questions about our bodies. Conventional medicine subordinates our subjective knowing, emphasizing that the ability to heal is not an innate human capacity but a result of medical training and techniques. We are taught that normal processes such as birth, menopause, and death are processes that require medical supervision and intervention. It is not encouraged, or even acknowledged, that we have the ability to be healthy without constant medical assistance. We learn that fatigue, hunger, sadness, stress, headaches, menstrual cramps, the sensations of childbirth, and most other physical feelings that are uncomfortable or unpleasant can be suppressed. We are not taught that these feelings are the language of our bodies, and that our bodies speak to us more and more strongly until we are finally forced to sit up and listen. This happens usually when we ignore little messages until they turn into discomforts, then symptoms, then outright diseases. But we can change this conditioning by listening to our bodies.

## Learning to Listen to Your Body

Each of us receives hundreds of messages from our body each day, informing us when, what, and how much to eat, when to sleep, when we need exercise, when to have a bowel movement, and so on. Your body is quick to detect when you are nourishing yourself and when you are harming yourself. This is true about not only the foods and substances that you ingest, but also the situations in which you find yourself, and the thoughts and feelings that you have. You can feel these responses, if you pay attention, in your nerves and muscles. For example, you may find that areas of your body tense up when you are in a stressful situation or that you sneeze in a room where a cat has recently been, if you are allergic to cats.

The concept of being body centered is not meant to imply separation of the body, mind, and emotions. In fact, all of these faculties are inextricably connected and interwoven in the organism we call a human being. On a literal and biological level, one cannot say that the mind begins here and ends there, as if the mind were only the brain, and the body everything below the brain. Actually, nerve pathways, hormones, and neurochemical messages course throughout the body, connecting the messages of the brain and body. Feelings occur when internal, physiological processes trigger various emotional responses as well as when external situations trigger biological and emotional reactions.

Being body centered means listening to your body when it's talking to you—and responding. You can learn to override and transform the culturally imposed and inauthentic voices that tell you how you should think and how you should be so that you know and accept who and how you truly are.

We would all benefit from listening to our bodies, and ideally we learn this skill prior to pregnancy. However, if you are new to this idea, pregnancy is a particularly ripe time for learning to listen because it is a time when your body manifests many new and noticeable messages.

Learning to listen to your body, like learning any language, takes time, commitment, and practice. People who are fluent in numerous languages often comment that the best way to learn a new language is to be totally immersed in hearing it, such as by spending time in a foreign country or at least by surrounding oneself with native speakers of that language. Pregnancy, though not separate from the continuity of a woman's life, is a unique experience permitting a time of total immersion in the language of the body, especially given many heightened physical sensations. Women are also apt to speak more freely with one another about their bodies when they are pregnant than they are at any other time, providing you with an opportunity to be around other women who are also trying to understand the language of their own bodies. Women who have already had children, "native speakers" if you will, are often eager to share their experiences. Spending time with women who have had natural and healthy experiences may help you gain comfort and confidence in listening to the unique language of your own body.

Pregnant women not only experience dramatic physical transformations, but also emotional and social transformations as our perceptions of ourselves as mothers grow and as our social roles and responsibilities change. However, unless we reflect about our attitudes toward our bodies and make a commitment to loving and trusting our bodies, we run the risk of carrying harmful patterns into our pregnancies. For example, a woman with an eating disorder may not allow herself and her baby to gain enough weight to nurture herself and her baby for a healthy pregnancy, birth, and postpartum. A woman who feels she is fat or not beautiful may become very depressed when her body is getting bigger as pregnancy progresses. This depression, unpleasant in itself, can also lead to physical problems such as poor dietary habits, bad posture constipation, or lower backache. This is just a simple example of how poor self-image, possibly based on comparing oneself to a cultural ideal, may be harmful during pregnancy.

Perhaps the most practical way to begin listening to your body is to pay attention to the most common messages you receive daily: hunger, thirst, fatigue, and need for elimination. Try to notice when you begin to feel the sensations that alert you to eat, drink, rest, or go to the bathroom. What are these sensations? When do you notice them? And most important, how do you respond to them?

- Do you eat when you're hungry, or do you think about whether you should eat and then skip a meal, afraid that if you eat too much you might get fat?

- Do you urinate when you feel the urge to, or like so many women, do you wait until a more convenient time or until you just can't wait any longer? Many women do the latter, not realizing that this can cause urinary tract infections, to which women are especially susceptible during pregnancy.

- Do you allow yourself to rest or sleep when you feel fatigued, or do you keep pushing yourself to do more until you collapse at the end of the day? Or do you push your body further with the help of coffee, chocolate, or sugar? Do you get down on yourself for being tired, thinking that you should be getting more done?

- Do you recognize that you may be feeling weepy, irritable, nauseated, faint, cold, and clammy, or that you have a headache because your blood sugar is too low and you need to eat a solid meal?

- Did you know that particular food cravings are your body's way of calling out for specific nutrients? For example, you may be craving sweets because you need more energy, but your body really needs more protein, which will provide you with more lasting energy.

Like many women, you may realize that you are not listening to your body. Just by deciding to be more alert to your own needs, you'll find yourself recognizing and responding to your body's signals more readily, and you will feel better for doing so. Keeping a journal can be a useful method for charting specific urges or sensations, as well as your responses and reactions. Remember that it takes time and patience to learn any language, but that you and your baby both deserve optimal care and loving attention.

# Feelings and Fears About Your Body

Another aspect of being body centered is to admit to yourself how you truly feel about your body. If you stand before a mirror unclothed, do you find yourself criticizing parts of your body? Do you criticize your nose, breasts, thighs, or buttocks? Try to understand where those critical messages came from—were you criticized as a child or as a teenager by other kids, or do you compare yourself to the images on magazine covers? Try to replace those old, critical voices with positive messages called "affirmations"—for example, "I love my body for growing my baby so well" or "I love these breasts, which will provide my baby with warm and nourishing milk." You can not only create a greater appreciation of your body by doing this but also actually improve your health by giving yourself positive affirmations about your inherently miraculous, beautiful, and unique self.

It is also helpful to acknowledge fears that you have about your body—for example, if you carry an undercurrent of fear that you won't be able to breastfeed or are afraid that your cervix won't dilate adequately in labor. All of us have heard stories of such problems, and sometimes we internalize other people's experiences. Being in a constant state of low-level fear can affect your health and thus indirectly increase the likelihood of a problem arising. If you harbor fears, or suspect you might, talk to your body in a loving way, saying something positive instead. Give yourself permission to accept and love your body just as it is, and trust that your body is perfectly designed for health. For example, if you fear that your cervix won't dilate adequately in labor, one of the things you can do is tell yourself daily, "My cervix will soften and open to birth my beautiful baby." You can visualize your cervix as a flower bud, gently and steadily opening, and you can put visual reminders of your opening cervix around your home: photographs of fully opened blossoms, or of the planet Saturn with its wide rings encircling the round planet much the way your cervix will eventually open around your baby's head.

*It's amazing what fears float around in our society about birth. At times, it takes a grand effort to swim past the worries. I try to stay focused on my love for my baby and my desire for him or her to be born in pure gentleness. In general, I have a deep and underlying faith in my body wisdom and the baby's as well.*

The basic idea is that if you have a negative body image, you can work actively to transform yourself into someone who feels genuinely good about herself and her abilities. You can use a journal for writing loving affirmations to your body. Expressive artwork, such as drawing, is also a way to create positive images for yourself.

From our earliest experiences, we are taught to squelch our emotions ("It's not nice to be angry," "Don't cry"—sometimes followed by "or I'll give you something to cry about"—or "You're a scaredy-cat") and to follow our rational minds.

We have also been taught that unpleasant physical sensations are a nuisance and encouraged to suppress such sensations with medication or by putting on a happy face. We were not taught that emotions are a signal of our comfort or discomfort in a given situation or environment and that our physical sensations let us know what is going on in our bodies. We were also never taught that our physical sensations can reflect our emotions. The best way to regain this knowledge is simply to stop and feel. If you have a headache coming on, you don't have to reach for the aspirin, or even herbs, nor do you have to analyze why you have a headache. By becoming very still and relaxed, and paying attention to your body from this still place, you will find that you can gain an awareness of exactly what you need to do for yourself—perhaps eat, drink water, rest, or remove yourself from a stressful situation. Perhaps an herbal remedy or speaking with a friend or health care provider will help. However, first you need to get in touch with that part of you that is your best authority. Try paying attention to how you feel emotionally about the sensations or discomforts you are having, and see what information you get from allowing yourself to feel your feelings. No one knows you better than you! One of the most important questions you can ask yourself several times each day is "What do I need right now?"

## Moving Your Body Joyously

Becoming body centered requires us to be oriented to our physical needs, and this includes spending time enjoying and nurturing our bodies. Bodies need to be moved, sometimes slowly and gracefully, sometimes quickly and with some force. Activities such as yoga, dance, swimming, walking briskly, volleyball, tennis, cross-country skiing, horseback riding, tai chi, you name it (as long as it is safe if you are already pregnant) are all ways to move your body joyously and exuberantly. They fill your body with vitality, stimulate your circulation (which improves cardiovascular functioning), oxygenate the body, enliven your mind, and lift and prevent depression. You not only improve your health and prepare your body for the very physical work of birth, but you also enrich your body awareness and self-esteem.

Receiving a regular massage is another way to get in touch with and nurture your body as you let tension melt away. In addition, massage is a form of passive exercise for the recipient, with many of the benefits of physical exercise, such as improved circulation and removal of waste products from the muscles. Scheduling problems and the high cost for professional massage need not prohibit you from exploring this possibility for nurturing your body. Your mate or a friend can give you a massage. Even as little as twenty minutes of massage on an occasional basis will be beneficial. (See chapter 7 for further discussions and explanations of both movement and massage techniques for pregnancy.)

As you learn to release tension from your body and develop appreciation and respect for it, you will gradually find yourself better able to respond to and nourish yourself. And you will discover that as you take better care of yourself, you will feel happier and healthier, and that your self-esteem and positive body image will come from within. You will like yourself just for being who you are.

## Reclaiming Women's Wisdom

*Women's wisdom* is a term used to encompass the practices and beliefs that women have developed over centuries and that still benefit women today—midwifery, nourishing and therapeutic methods of food preparation, herbalism, and healing touch, to name a few. Women have often been the primary physicians for families, tribes, and villages. These are the main healing modalities that I draw upon in this book.

Women's wisdom is also based on the stories that women tell about their lives and what we can learn from these stories. Women's wisdom allows us to bring our whole selves to our experience—including our feelings, intuition, and body wisdom along with our intellect—rather than fragmented parts of ourselves. Likewise, in women's ways of healing, there is the awareness that healing must occur in the person's life, not just in her body, and that physical healing alone cannot occur until the underlying factors of illness and discomfort are addressed. These factors may be as simple as finding more time in your own life, say thirty minutes twice a week, to nurture yourself in whatever way suits you, or as complex as a job or major relationship change!

Women's wisdom embraces our subjective knowledge drawn from feelings and personal experience. This intuition may include dreaming about your baby before conception and sensing who the child will be, as well as transpersonal knowing, such as having abdominal cramps only to discover that your best friend or sister is in early labor. These are all without logical explanation; they are sympathetic experiences that allow us to realize that there are mysterious aspects of our connection to our bodies and to each other.

These experiences remind us that there is more to life than meets the eye, and that there really is no separation between the mind, body, and spirit.

In myth and religion, women have historically been considered more closely related to the mysterious aspects of life than men because of our experiences of menstruation and pregnancy and our ability to birth our young. Modern intellectual reductionist culture has discredited this multisensory awareness, considering it unreliable, even nonexistent. Nevertheless, we value emotional and sensory experiences. Women have long recognized the deep psychic connections between a mother and child, knowing, for example, even from thousands of miles away, when a child is in danger. Breastfeeding mothers are all too familiar with the experience of having their breasts begin to leak milk while they are at work, only to find out later that their baby had awakened from a nap at the same time and was crying to be fed. This kind of intuitive awareness is too common to be dismissed as coincidental and too valuable for us to dismiss as fallacious.

Reclaiming women's wisdom restores value to intuition as *part* of our intelligence. We have to reclaim women's wisdom *and* proclaim that we are the true authorities of ourselves.

Learning to trust and recognize our intuition and body messages is particularly valuable for pregnant women. Pregnancy is a time when you and your baby are experiencing many increased nutritional demands as well as a greater need for nourishment in other areas, such as massage, exercise, rest, and relaxation. Our body awareness alerts us to our needs, and our intuition can help us to name exactly what we need to do to meet them. One example of using intuitive guidance occurred with a very young couple, with whom I worked long ago, who were

---

### Your *Yoni*

One of the ways that I and other women have chosen to reclaim what is rightfully ours is to replace the word *vagina* with the word *yoni*. *Vagina* literally means a "sheath," and is obviously a reference to the idea that our sexual organs exist only in relationship to men's needs. *Yoni*, however, is a Sanskrit word for the female genitalia and refers to the sacredness of a woman's sexual self. In this book you will often see the word *yoni* used where you might commonly use the word *vagina*.

---

having their first baby. The woman, actually still a teenager, had a very poor diet, consisting in large part of pizza and candy bars. I felt that she needed to recognize what her body told her she needed to eat. I taught her and her partner the following exercise: I had them sit facing each other, holding hands. I suggested they ask the baby what he or she needed right now for optimal nourishment. They were both completely silent for a few moments, waiting for a response from the baby. When they both became quite still, I told them to open their eyes and voice what they heard. Simultaneously, both the father and the mother said, "Carrots, the baby needs more carrots." So the mother ate more carrots, practiced this exercise more often, improved her diet greatly, and gave birth at home very easily (after a three-hour labor) to a healthy baby.

Today, as we try to ensure the healthy development of our babies during pregnancy, we can look beyond the conventional prenatal care offered by a typical obstetrician. Exploring your intuitive connection with your baby and trusting your inner wisdom can help you grow a healthy baby.

As you explore the various healing options available for supporting pregnancy health, I invite you to reacquaint yourself with your women's wisdom and discover the techniques that can best nourish you, your baby, and your family.

# CHAPTER 3

# The Baby Inside You

*The first moment of* awareness that you are pregnant is profound—for many women profoundly joyful, for most women overwhelming, and for some, not such a welcome realization.

I knew as soon as I conceived. My breasts ached. I started peeing more. But something else and more subtle felt different. My dreams become more vivid. I became more sensitive.

With my second, I had vivid dreams of seeing a magnificent seashell in the ocean, too deep for me to reach, so my husband dove for it. The shell he handed me had a deep pink, shimmering lining that in waking consciousness reminded me of my womb's lining. At my third child's conception, my husband and I felt a breeze come over us, as if a door had opened, and with my fourth baby, somehow I just knew she was with me. Once I realized I was pregnant, I also had concerns about my baby's well-being, eating well enough, and making sure I was avoiding anything that could be harmful to my baby.

## Your Growing Baby

The intention of this chapter is to facilitate your inner awareness of your baby. As a midwife, I am so aware of feeling babies' arms, legs, little bottoms, and heads while they are still in their mamas' wombs, that a baby in the womb is almost as tangible to me as a baby in arms. However, and especially if this is your first baby, it may seem a bit intangible that there's a person inside there. Having a clear visual idea of how babies generally develop can help you to make the conscious connection with your baby more real.

Pregnancy begins at the time of conception but is dated from the time of the first day of your last menstrual period (LMP). Pregnancy is considered to be forty-two weeks long, counting the two weeks between your period and conception, or about forty weeks until the baby is fully "cooked." The information below is based on a baby's age since conception. If you want a general idea of what stage of growth your baby is in at, say, six weeks, read about the development at both five and seven weeks too.

## CONCEPTION

Pregnancy begins at conception when the sperm and ovum unite. This brings both parents' genetic potential into contact and creates the physical foundation of a new life—your baby. Fertilization generally occurs in the fallopian tube and then over the next five days, as the *zygote* divides into a cluster comprised of numerous cells, it makes its way toward the uterus, where, by about the sixth day, it attaches to the uterine lining. The process of implantation is complete by about the tenth or eleventh day after conception. By the end of the first two weeks, placental formation has begun and the cells of the baby are beginning to differentiate. The first two weeks are known as the *preembryonic* phase.

## WEEKS THREE THROUGH SEVEN

From week three through seven after conception, the developing baby is referred to as an *embryo*. It is during this remarkable period of development that all of the baby's essential features and body parts will be formed. Because it is the most vulnerable phase of development for the baby, it is important for pregnant women to avoid all substances such as alcohol and drugs (including many prescription and over-the-counter medications), and environmental contaminants, such as pesticides, chemical fumes, and cigarette smoke, that could harm the baby.

By the fifteenth day after conception, when you might be expecting your period to start, you may notice breast tenderness and a feeling of fullness in your abdomen. This is the way you would normally feel before your period. If you tried to conceive, you may have already begun to take special care of yourself even before you missed your period. If your period is late, then it is sensible to treat yourself as if you were pregnant until it is clear whether or not you are. This will afford your baby optimal protection for healthy development.

During week three, the shape of the baby begins to take form.

In the fourth week, the heart begins beating, and by the end of this week, the embryo has assumed the appearance of a salamander. There are arm and leg buds, facial and neck structures, and small pits that will later become the ears. By the end of this week, your baby is less than a ¼-inch long.

The fifth week brings extensive growth of the brain and head and the beginning development of the eyes. Because a baby's growth occurs from top to bottom, the head is large in relation to the body.

During the sixth week after conception, the nose, mouth, and palate take shape, and the eyelids form. By this time, the arms and legs have developed rapidly so that by the seventh week, the baby has clearly defined wrists, elbows, knees, fingers, toes, and so on. The baby is now about half an inch long.

In the seventh week, the baby's urogenital system is developing, the neck area is established, and the external ears are visible. By the end of this week, the baby clearly looks like a human baby. The end of the seventh week is also the end of what is called the *embryonic* period.

At this point, all of the baby's essential structures, both internal and external, have been formed and require only further growth and development. By now, the baby can respond to touch: if it were possible to touch the baby's palm, the baby's hand would close. The baby can touch his or her own face as well as make other gentle movements.

## WEEK TEN

At ten weeks, the baby begins to have both hair and fingernails and it's possible to differentiate boys from girls.

## WEEK TWELVE

By twelve weeks, the baby is about 3¾ inches long and weighs about an ounce. The baby is able to make facial expressions and has lips that can make sucking motions. In fact, the baby can now swallow amniotic fluid and pee it out, too. The eyes are almost fully developed and the lids fused closed while the rest of this development occurs. By this time, your uterus is about the size of a large grapefruit and you are already entering the second trimester of your pregnancy. If you have been nauseated and uncomfortable, you will soon begin to feel much better.

## WEEK FOURTEEN

At fourteen weeks, the baby is covered with *lanugo*, downy hair that grows in whorls over the body. The baby has fingerprints, nipples appear, and the back, which has been curved, straightens. The bones are hardening, and the baby, who fills your womb, is now becoming more active. You may even notice movement, particularly when you are resting.

## WEEK SIXTEEN
By sixteen weeks, the baby measures 7 or 8 inches in length and weighs about 4 ounces.

## MONTH FIVE
At five months, the legs reach their full length and toenails form. By now, you are likely to notice some subtle fluttering movements or even some obvious "kicks and pokes." If you've not yet noticed movement, it is likely that you will soon. The baby also hiccups occasionally, which you will feel as a series of rhythmic "knocks" in your belly. Your baby can suck his or her thumb, grasp the umbilical cord, and even scratch his or her face. There is more hair on the head, and eyebrows are formed. The eyes are still fused shut. The body is now covered with *vernix* (which literally translates as "cheese"), a creamy substance that protects the baby's skin from the surrounding water. The heartbeat may now be audible by fetoscope and will usually range between 120 and 160 beats per minute. The baby's ears are now fully functional, and because water conducts sound so well (when we are underwater sounds are muffled because we have air in our ears, but babies have no air in theirs while in the womb), the baby hears sounds all of the time—the rhythms of your heart and breath, the placenta, and your digestion, as well as all of your speaking, singing, crying, yelling, praying, and so on. The baby is able to hear and respond to music and will also respond to your emotions with more or less gentle movements. It is therefore optimal to surround yourself with beautiful and soothing music as well as to make your own sounds as peaceful, joyous, and comforting as possible. Through sound, the baby begins to learn about the world. Your baby is now about 10 or 12 inches long and weighs about 8 ounces.

## MONTH SIX
At six months, the skin is wrinkled, translucent, and appears red, due to the blood being visible through the skin. Permanent tooth buds are present, and hair growth is obvious. The eyes open, and the baby can make both crying and sucking motions. Strong arm and leg muscles have developed, and if the foot is tickled, the baby will respond by planting the foot downward. You may notice that the baby responds to your touch with movements. The baby is 12 to 14 inches long and weighs about 1$^{1}/_{2}$ pounds.

## MONTH SEVEN

At seven months, the lungs, though not fully mature, could function minimally outside the uterus. The baby would have a good chance of survival if born prematurely at this point. The baby now sees sunlight through your abdomen and will turn away from very bright light. He or she is about 15 inches long and weighs 3 to 4 pounds. The baby will gain about a half pound a week.

## MONTH EIGHT

During the eighth month, the baby begins to put on fat and the wrinkled skin begins to smooth out. Vernix and lanugo still cover the baby, except for the face, but these will gradually lessen in quantity by birth. The baby is between 16 and 18 inches long and may weigh between 4 and 7 pounds.

20 Weeks

24 Weeks

28 Weeks

32 Weeks

36 Weeks

40 Weeks

## MONTH NINE

At nine months, the lanugo and vernix have begun to disappear, and the baby is reaching full maturity, ready for life outside of your womb. All of the sense organs are well formed, and the rest of the organs are ready for extrauterine life. The wrinkles have disappeared, and the baby's head will begin to settle into your pelvis, ready for birth. The baby is now 19 to 21 inches long and on the average weighs between 6 and 9 pounds.

# Creating a Healthy Prenatal Environment

During pregnancy, you are quite literally your child's environment. Constantly emerging data makes it clear that lifelong health begins in the mom's womb. Chemicals in our environments, the foods we eat—even our moods and stress levels—can have an impact on whether our child grows up with or eventually develops allergies, asthma, eczema, colic, autism, diabetes—even cancer. Wow—this is a huge amount of responsibility!

Unfortunately, these days, pregnant mommas are faced with a whole new set of quite realistic concerns about the harmful things to which most of us *are* exposed to in our environment. Just yesterday, for example, I received a medical journal article with the title "Does Cancer Start in the Womb? Altered Mammary Gland Development and Predisposition to Breast Cancer Due to in Utero Exposure to Endocrine Disruptors."

While I'd love to simply reassure you and say don't worry, the reality is that our environment is filled with many "new to nature" chemicals and environmental contaminants that our bodies have no idea how to use, process, and eliminate. Sadly, we do need to have a high level of concern for what we are exposed to during pregnancy.

*We can nourish our babies so that they may enjoy prenatal wellness and be prepared to meet the inevitable challenges of the world.*

Not too long ago, it was believed that the placenta protected babies in the womb from chemicals to which the mom might be exposed. But a study by the Environmental Working Group (EWG) in collaboration with Commonweal, found an average of two hundred industrial chemicals and pollutants (including consumer product ingredients and wastes from burning coal, gasoline, and garbage) in umbilical cord blood from a random selection of babies born in U.S. hospitals.

It is now known that both baby and mom are awash in a sea of chemical exposures. And most frightening is that we have no idea what impact this chemical stew is having on our bodies. We know that a developing baby's chemical exposures are greater pound for pound than those of adults and that these chemicals have a more profound impact on the developing brain and organs. Further, physiological systems that naturally detoxify chemicals are still immature in the developing baby, thus toxins may linger longer or have a more detrimental impact than on adults.

There is solid evidence that not only does cancer potentially start in the womb, but so can asthma, birth defects, diabetes, heart disease, depression, and a host of other lifelong chronic medical problems. The good news is that there are simple and reliable steps you can take to maximize your baby's health even before birth and avoid as many of these exposures as possible.

## EAT ORGANIC AND AVOID HIGH-MERCURY FISH

While the nutritional value of organic foods over conventional has recently been debated, there is no question that organic is better for your body and the environment from a chemical-exposures perspective. And exposure to agricultural chemicals in utero can cause long-term health consequences.

The great news is that studies have clearly demonstrated that even just a few days of eating organic foods significantly reduces the blood levels of harmful chemicals—and staying on organics is likely to keep them lower than eating a conventional-foods diet.

Whether to eat organic only is a cost issue for many of us. To learn which foods are organic "musts," visit the Environmental Working Group website and focus on avoiding what are called the "dirty dozen" foods and emphasize eating the "clean 15," which are products that do not have significant amounts of pesticide residues. Because the fats in dairy and meat are repositories for environmental chemicals, buying these organically (or from antibiotic- and hormone-free sources) is important for protecting baby.

In addition to eating organic, pregnant women will want to avoid fish that are high in mercury, which can cause neurological problems in the developing fetus. These include tuna, shark, swordfish, king mackerel, tilefish, sea bass, Gulf Coast oysters, marlin, halibut, pike, walleye, and largemouth bass. I recommend no more than two servings of fish per week—and no high-mercury fish at all during pregnancy (or preferably ever, for that matter!).

## AVOID ENDOCRINE DISRUPTORS AND
## COMMON ENVIRONMENTAL TOXINS

Excellent data shows that a pregnant woman's exposure to a variety of environmental toxins—ranging from bisphenol A (BPA), found in many food packages and plastics, to heavy metals—can have deleterious effects on the baby. We know that environmental chemicals called endocrine disruptors mimic hormones and are associated with problems such as genital birth defects in baby boys, for example, hypospadias, as well as later development of diabetes in children and adults.

I encourage all pregnant women to avoid foods that come in soft plastic wrap, to avoid heating or microwaving foods in plastic containers, and to use glass storage containers and drink only out of glass water bottles rather than plastic ones.

Body products, including many cosmetics, may also contain a variety of toxins and heavy metals. Lead has been found in many brands of lipstick! Household cleaning products can also be sources of toxic exposures.

Going green is a sure way to reduce your baby's prenatal exposures to a host of toxins. And of course, avoid the obvious exposures, like smoking, drugs, and anything more than the most modest amount of alcohol and that only after the first trimester.

While we cannot control everything in our environment, we can do a great deal to minimize exposures and impact—and with nutrition—as you will read about later.

## REDUCE STRESS

Stress is sort of a fact of life for pretty much everyone. Normal amounts of day-to-day stress—you know, feeling exhausted because of taking care of your other kids, balancing work and home life, normal concerns about pregnancy—are just par for the course of living. But sustained stress can affect your baby in three ways—the first is that we don't take optimal care of ourselves when we're stressed. We tend to skimp on nutrition, exercise, and sleep—so baby might not be getting our best. Second, stress hormones, when sustained, can affect the baby's internal chemical environment—setting the baby up for anxiety or depression later in life. And third, stress hormones can affect oxygen as well as blood flow to the baby. Thus relaxing and getting the stressors out of your life are almost as important as getting good nutrition! Learning meditation and relaxation techniques now can also give you some super helpful tools to have on hand for long nights with a teething baby or long car rides with a cranky toddler.

Depression in pregnancy is a bit of a complicated topic. The conventional wisdom until recently has been that the effect of untreated depression in the mom can have devastating impacts on the baby, particularly after birth when depression in mom can lead to neglect of baby. As a result, treatment with antidepressants in pregnancy has been commonplace and has been thought to be generally safe or at least worth the risk that they were less of a problem than the risk of not treating the depression with medication. Now there is concern that antidepressant use by a pregnant mom can actually lead to problems ranging from cardiac defects to autism. Yet the risks of untreated depression remain.

Nutrition, vitamin and mineral supplementation, and some herbs have great promise in treating depression, especially when combined with effective therapy and optimal social support whether through your partner, family, friends, or a pregnancy group.

## Communicating with Your Baby

Moms and babies have a literal cellular connection. A lot of my clients don't let themselves bond with their babies until they get ultrasound or first trimester screening confirmation that baby is healthy. Of course fear of loss is understandable. But a real connection can be fostered even without seeing baby on a screen, knowing whether the baby is a boy or a girl, or hearing the baby's heartbeat.

While it is true that you may feel more confident in your pregnancy after receiving some objective measure of your health or the baby's health via a prenatal diagnostic test (keeping in mind that many tests of fetal well-being are inaccurate), you will have to decide for yourself at what point you draw the line between a natural experience and a technological experience. Therefore, it is up to you to be well informed as to the benefits, risks, and necessity of such testing, and to choose for yourself what you do and don't want done. Developing a strong prenatal connection with your baby, as well as trusting in your inner knowing, will enable you to make the most appropriate use of technology during birth, your child's early years, and possibly later.

Communicating with your baby, as with anyone, is a two-way exchange—that is, you can communicate with your baby and he or she can communicate with you. It is quite possible for this communication to begin even before pregnancy occurs through dreams and extrasensory awareness. For example, before I conceived my second child, I had a vivid dream, which I recorded in my journal, of being in a snowstorm with a close woman friend. In the dream, she went into a room and I assisted her at the birth of her child, a girl, and then I went into an adjacent room and birthed my own baby, also a girl. Several months after this dream, my friend conceived a baby, and in the following month I too conceived. Later I assisted her—in the midst of a snowstorm—at the birth of her daughter, and weeks later I birthed my baby, also a daughter.

## TALKING TO YOUR BABY

Throughout your pregnancy, talk to the baby during your day, sharing even mundane tasks, the music you love, your musings about the beauty of the world around you. Massage your baby during the day by rubbing and patting your belly and also each morning when you rise or each evening before you sleep. During these relaxed times, put a little oil on your hands and rub deeply, actually massaging the parts of the baby's body that you feel. This cannot hurt your baby, and babies respond positively to such caring during the pregnancy as well as after the birth with excellent growth. Babies that have been regularly massaged prenatally will love to be massaged throughout childhood. This is an excellent technique for the prevention of illness as well as a remedial treatment. Talk to your baby as you massage her or his body, or sing a special, beautiful song. Chances are the baby will continue to be soothed by this song after birth and will quickly learn to sing it once she or he learns to speak.

Some mothers enjoy reading verses of poetry or children's books to their babies even before birth. These books will probably become your child's all-time favorites, as babies definitely have exhibited preferences from their prenatal time.

Speaking affirmations to your child can foster your confidence as well as nourish the baby's growth with ideas that reinforce his or her well-being. For example, as you massage your baby, you can repeat a few times, rhythmically, "You are so welcome and wanted here; we love you so" or "You are a strong and healthy baby" or "I welcome you for whoever you are." These positive statements can also be used to help you dispel anxieties that may creep into your mind about the baby's health or normal development. As you get closer to the birth, you can say things like "We are so ready for you to be born; we welcome you into our open arms" or "It is safe to be born, and we look forward to holding and caring for you, dear baby."

## LISTENING TO YOUR BABY

Each day when you take time to quietly rub your baby, become silent and ask your baby, "What do you need?" Ask if there is anything the baby wants you to know. Then just listen very quietly and you may be surprised at what you hear. You may not hear a baby's "voice," but in time you may feel a message coming through to you.

Many pregnant women have disturbing dreams—for example, that baby is deformed. Try not to take these literally (if mine were literal my son would have been a litter of seven black Labrador retriever puppies instead of a cute little boy!). Dreams are a landscape that let you work out and explore your fears and anxieties. If you have particularly disturbing dreams, discuss this with your midwife—she can help you to process your worries and might even have a logical explanation— for example, that you are eating something that is disturbing your sleep!

## INVITING CREATIVE INSIGHTS

Keeping a journal of your insights or dreams about your baby or memorable things that happened during the pregnancy is a great way to build a living history that your child can later look back on and enjoy with you. Make a note of the words to the songs you sing, stories you read to the baby, or particularly magical places you visit during your pregnancy.

One of my favorite forms of receiving insight about my baby is through artwork. I'm not a professional artist, but I do enjoy the experience of creating, so I'll sit down with blank paper and supplies and let my body talk through whatever medium I am using. I find that colored chalks and oil pastels reflect the subtle energy of pregnancy since the lines and colors can be blended to create a smooth, soft image. Many supplies are available inexpensively at art supply stores; you can therefore enjoy yourself without spending a fortune. It is best to avoid art supplies that contain toxic metals (as do many oil paints) and those with strong fumes. Acrylic paints, most watercolor paints, pastels, colored pencils, and chalks are safe for use during pregnancy.

I've found myself creating images of wings surrounding babies, mothers holding babies, buds opening, and so on. Let your body speak to you. Go deep within yourself to find the reservoir of creativity and intuition, and express yourself from there. Artwork can open and release blocked creative energy and be highly therapeutic, but only if you do it for enjoyment and don't judge your results.

The joyous welcoming of your child into your life sends messages to your child that will help him or her to thrive. None of us can be happy 100 percent of the time, but we can choose to stay in close touch with the messages we are sending our babies. How we treat them prenatally can set the tone for how they will treat themselves and expect others to treat them for much of their lives. While prenatal influences are not the only influences that emboss patterns on our psyches and emotions, they do hold great sway over us. We can help a whole generation of children to feel loved. This will sow the seeds of loving each other and creating a just world coming from our most evolved awareness.

*If you listen to your baby and be very quiet, you may "hear" your baby telling you something important.*

# CHAPTER 4

# Prenatal Care

>>>>><<<<<

*When most people refer* to prenatal care, they mean prenatal medical monitoring. Focused almost exclusively on detecting and reducing medical problems such as premature delivery, birth defects, and infant mortality, conventional prenatal care neglects to place adequate emphasis on nutrition, exercise, and emotional, social, and psychological health, all of which are essential to the optimal health of mothers and babies. To improve prenatal care in this country, we need to place more emphasis on ensuring that all women have access to healthy foods, reduced stress, and other necessities of prenatal health rather than narrowly directing our resources to the research and development of sophisticated methods of prenatal testing. An ultrasound cannot help a baby grow—food does!

The most significant prenatal care you will receive is the care you give to yourself. Ideally, this is what the additional prenatal care you get from a health care provider will nurture. And the key to excellent prenatal care is individual care rather than routine procedures applied universally to all women.

Prenatal care also includes pampering yourself a bit—making sure the people around you are good people for you to be spending time with, setting limits for when you need some downtime from household responsibilities and older kids if you have them, letting your partner give you a back rub or leg massage—or getting a professional massage now and then if you can't get a massage at home.

# Prenatal Care Basics

The purpose of prenatal care is to support your health on multiple levels (physically, mentally, emotionally), maximize the potential for your baby's health, and foster the health of your growing family so you are prepared during pregnancy for the birth, and beyond as well.

An ideal care provider is:

- Sensitive to your needs and the changing needs of your family

- Knowledgeable about optimal nutrition, exercise, and mental and emotional well-being

- Knowledgeable about and skilled in addressing the medical issues that can arise in pregnancy and birth

- Sensitive, considerate, responsible, and professional, yet warm

- Able to help you become educated, well informed, and confident about your body

She must also maintain excellent relationships with other health care practitioners so that she can help the mother receive the care she requires. Midwives are the most likely to fit this bill!

I refer to prenatal care providers as women throughout this book because I believe that women are the most appropriate care providers for pregnant women. While there are sensitive male obstetricians and male nurse-midwives, I strongly believe that it is women's rightful place to provide prenatal and birth care. This is how it has been throughout history until the recent past, and this is how I believe it should be again. However, many women still take comfort in a male physician. If you do choose a male care provider, choose one who truly respects women.

Most practitioners (obstetricians, certified nurse-midwives, or traditional midwives, certified or not) see pregnant women on generally the same prenatal schedule, once a month until thirty-two weeks of pregnancy, then bimonthly until thirty-six weeks, then weekly until the birth. Many of the same procedures are done—for example, determining the position of the baby, checking blood pressure, and so on (see "Prenatal Visits" later in this chapter). However, the way a practitioner has been trained greatly affects her or his philosophies and perspectives, and thus, your care. This section provides an overview of the main types of care providers currently in the United States. Of course, these descriptions are generalizations, and any practitioner may be more or less holistically or medically oriented. You will have to decide which approach you are looking for and then choose an appropriate care provider. Happily, many practitioners offer a free consultation, which can help you make choices that are right for you.

## Choosing Your Birth Place

Most women prefer to birth in the hospital because of perceived levels of greater safety. While hospitals do afford quick and ready access to emergency services, and are the appropriate place for women with pregnancy or anticipated birth complications or need for *operative birth* (cesarean section), hospitals are also not benign places for birth.

Routine hospital procedures and policies such as not eating during labor, use of continuous external fetal monitoring, regular vaginal exams, and use of medications such as Pitocin and epidurals during labor increase your risk of developing problems in labor and birth as well as the risk of infection, cesarean section, and numerous associated problems.

Birthing centers, whether in the hospital or free standing, can be a nice middle ground if you want to have a more homelike environment than most hospitals provide. If the birthing center is associated with and close to a hospital, you can often still have fairly quick access to emergency medical care should the need arise; however, your "birth plan" if you have one, may be curtailed by whatever guidelines and regulations the hospital or birthing center dictate. If you choose a birthing center that lacks hospital affiliation, you may mistakenly believe that being in a birthing center is affording you medical security; however, many are simply run by midwives and offer no more medical protection than a home birth, so know which type of birthing center you are choosing if having access to emergency medical services is on your list.

Home birth is an option for women who are in excellent health and have low-risk pregnancies. They are largely attended by midwives. A rare few obstetricians and family doctors attend home births, but those that do can provide you with excellent options and seamless transport between home and hospital.

Home births may be attended by a variety of types of midwives ranging from graduate school level–trained CNMs to licensed nonnurse midwives to religiously or philosophically self-proclaimed midwives. So knowing what you're looking for

*It's like growing food—if you take care of the soil, the food will grow. Cluck over the mother, nurture her.*

—CANDACE FIELDS-WHITRIDGE, CNM

and who you're getting is really important. Midwives (with occasional assistance from a physician or nurse-midwife) have been fighting the battle to keep alive the right to birth at home with a skilled attendant. This right to birth at home has been challenged in most states, to the point that many midwives have been arrested or harassed. While I cannot discuss this issue at length in this book, I encourage you to read books such as *The American Way of Birth* by Jessica Mitford and *Immaculate Deception* by Suzanne Arms, as well as other titles in the Bibliography (page 271). For a complete discussion of the statistics on midwifery and home birth safety as well as the process of choosing a care provider and birth setting, you might wish to consult my book *A Pocket Guide to Midwifery Care*.

## Choosing Your Birth Attendant

In the United States, midwives are the lead maternity care providers for 8 to 9 percent of women during pregnancy and childbirth, family physicians are the lead maternity care providers for 6 to 7 percent of women, and obstetrician-gynecologists care for most of the remainder. Women birth more easily and with fewer complications when attended by a supportive woman—a friend, relative, or doula (a woman trained in the support of laboring women, and hired for this purpose). However, even with a doula, it is ideal when you feel comfortable, open, and relaxed with whomever is going to work with you to get that baby born! After all, birth is about being able to be open!

*Care that is provided by another woman can be special. A midwife is a birthing woman's equal, not her authority. She is a confidante. She understands the importance of being respectful and gentle with another person's most intimate parts of herself. She knows that safety in childbirth is more a matter of prevention than treatment, of listening closely, helping a woman have a healthy attitude, and promoting normalcy. She protects both the privacy of the woman and the integrity of the family.*

—ELIZABETH DAVIS,
*Heart and Hands: A Midwife's Guide to Pregnancy and Birth*

Where you choose to have your baby will have an influence on who your care provider will be. If you are choosing a hospital birth, your options include obstetricians, family physicians, and midwives. Most birthing center births and hospital births are attended by certified nurse midwives (CNM), who have attended nursing school then subsequently completed three years of graduate nursing education in the care of women during pregnancy and birth, as well as in general well-woman care. Direct-entry midwives, those who have become midwives either through a variety of accredited and nonaccredited schools or apprenticeship without first becoming nurses, are also licensed in many states and may attend birthing center or even hospital births in some of these.

## OBSTETRICIANS

Obstetricians are physicians who, in addition to their four years of medical training, have trained for four additional years in obstetrics and gynecology, preparing them to assist women through both normal and complicated pregnancies and births. They are trained to provide women with gynecological care from puberty through old age. Pregnancy and birth are seen as medical events. Few obstetricians are trained to let the mother be the orchestrator of her own health care and, because of their training, may come to see all pregnant women as emergencies waiting to happen. Further, many go into obstetrics out of a love for surgery. Thus it should be no surprise, given fear of birth and love of surgery, that we have a national cesarean section rate that exceeds 33 percent! Obstetric care is strongly influenced by medical legal considerations, with the average obstetrician expecting to be sued at least three times in her career; therefore, in the interest of legal self-protection, many obstetricians use routine protocols with all patients. Overwhelmingly, obstetricians require that patients give birth in a hospital setting. However, some obstetricians will help women achieve natural births in the hospital. A few courageous obstetricians do have home-birth practices.

Obstetrical care may be best for those women with a high likelihood of developing complications during pregnancy or birth, such as those with diabetes, kidney or heart disease, eclampsia, hypertension, or any problem that is likely to require medical intervention or emergency care. Obstetric care, when compared with midwifery care, is much more likely to lead to medical intervention in labor and birth.

Here are some questions to ask an obstetrician you are interviewing:

- What is your cesarean rate?

- What is your episiotomy rate?

- What is the rate of induced births in your practice?

- How many women in your practice breastfeed their babies?

- What are your feelings about natural birth?

- What are your philosophies about birth?

- How much time do you spend with women at prenatal visits?

- Will you be at my birth or will another physician attend (and if so, who will that be)?

- What are your policies for women who go past-due, who have had previous cesarean sections, for permitted length of labor and pushing?

- Do you encourage women to participate actively in prenatal care and the birth?

## FAMILY PHYSICIANS

Family physicians trained with a specialty in obstetrics go through the same medical training as obstetricians and then do a residency that includes comprehensive obstetrics and gynecology, however, with less gynecologic surgical training than obstetricians. Some family physicians have the same privileges and rights, including permission to do cesarean sections and other surgery, as obstetricians. Some choose to practice low-risk obstetrics, and if complications arise in pregnancy or birth, transfer care to an obstetrician or maternal fetal medicine specialist. Family medicine training tends to be more about preventing problems than intervening in a natural process, and family physicians are more likely to be open-minded about natural approaches to childbirth. However, they are obligated to the same standards of care that guide obstetricians and hospital births. As with obstetricians, some family doctors work in birthing centers and a rare few attend or support home births.

## MIDWIVES

Midwives embody a philosophy that honors the importance of the pregnant woman in the entire childbearing experience. At all times, the woman is treated with respect and sensitivity for the intelligent adult that she is. Midwives also maintain respect and sensitivity for the needs of the baby. Perhaps the central belief that unites midwives is that pregnancy and birth are natural processes for which women are inherently and biologically capable, and that, with the participation of the woman in caring for herself and with the assistance and guidance of the midwife, the woman will enjoy a healthy experience. Midwives honor childbearing as a rite of passage and therefore encourage full participation by the mother during pregnancy and birth, and support her in this transition, helping her to grow in confidence and ability to nurture herself and her baby both before and after birth.

Good-quality midwifery care has been demonstrated to be associated with lower rates of medical complications and birth interventions, as well as greater client satisfaction, compared with conventional obstetrics. Many of the innovations and progressive changes that have occurred in hospitals in recent years have been inspired by the kind of intimate, professional care provided by midwives.

But not all midwives are created equal, so it is important to consider what your needs are and what different midwives have to offer you and your baby in terms of education, skill, and safety.

Nurse-midwives have completed the same training as registered nurses, and then have additionally specialized in midwifery care through three years of graduate school training. Nurse midwives offer many distinct advantages as birth attendants: they possess a recognized level of training and because of their licensing, are able to practice in home, birthing center, and hospital settings, and provide you with a balance of woman-centered care with an affinity for natural birth. They also offer medical testing, and when needed, a limited number of medical interventions, for example, starting an IV or administering medications for bleeding after birth. Many not only offer prenatal and birthing services, but can continue to see you for well-woman care over the years, providing Pap smears and birth control, for example. Most nurse-midwives are incredibly woman centered and are dedicated to keeping birth as natural as possible. Sometimes their training and licensure can be a deficit in that they are typically trained in the medical model and in a medical setting, so may have restrictions on how far they can go outside of the guidelines of what is medically defined as normal—even when they disagree with those guidelines. So, for example, you might be planning a wonderful birthing center or home birth with a midwife, but if she is obligated to transfer your care to a hospital or obstetrician if you are in labor for more than a certain amount of time, then this is just what she'll have to do. Also, their training may not include home birth, thus they may not be equipped to handle emergencies outside of the hospital or medical environment, and some may bring a more medical-management approach even to home birth, which may not be what you anticipated.

Certified professional midwives (CPMs) and licensed midwives (LMs) are direct-entry midwives, meaning that they entered the profession without first becoming nurses. CPM and LMs primarily attend home births, though in an increasing number of states, they may also practice in or even own or operate birthing centers or clinics where they provide prenatal care and birthing services.

In the United States, unlike in Europe, the training for direct-entry midwives is not standardized. CPMs are certified via the North American Registry of Midwives (NARM), an independent credentialing organization with core requirements for

> *Pregnancy is a great time to have sex—you can't get pregnant!*
>
> —INA MAY GASKIN

sitting a certification examination that must then be passed to earn that title. This exam is used by some states as the licensing exam for midwives in that state, and some states recognize the CPM credential for licensure. Licensure in some states may require that midwives attend a recognized school, but not all do. Training at a recognized school is not required for receipt of a CPM credential; NARM recognizes apprenticeship training. Most midwives train as apprentices under the tutelage of other experienced midwives, gaining extensive clinical experience by attending numerous women throughout pregnancy, birth, and afterward. Many receive excellent training through accredited schools and apprenticeships, but the quality of training can be inconsistent and one can be eligible to take the exam based on numbers of births attended rather than demonstrated quality of the learning environment.

In addition to CNMs, CPMs, and LMs, there are midwives who are trained in a variety of settings. They can range from being highly qualified to not qualified at all, have varying levels of knowledge, and have training that ranges from excellent to sorely insufficient.

Direct-entry midwives are often knowledgeable about traditional, folk, and natural methods of both preventing and treating problems that can arise during pregnancy, birth, and the postpartum period. This can be a tremendous asset in preserving the potential for natural birth, because often the less intervention there is during the birthing of a healthy pregnant woman, the greater the opportunity for the most natural birth.

On the other hand, not all direct-entry midwives are skilled and competent in the management of emergency complications, and while these are rare, these are the times you really need someone who knows what she's doing! To some women seeking a midwife, a midwife's skills at handling complications may be less significant than the personal relationship with that midwife. It is your birth, and if you choose a midwife with minimal experience because you feel that your relationship with her is the most important factor, that is your right; however, this choice must be based on honest information provided by your midwife, and it is your responsibility to arrange access to a practitioner or facility capable of handling an emergency should one arise beyond the capability of you or your practitioner. It is unfair to you and your baby, as well as your midwife, to expect her to be able to help you should an unexpected complication arise for which she lacks the necessary skills.

As with all professions, midwives vary in their skills and integrity. It is therefore up to you to determine the level of skill you want your midwife to possess (including the type of equipment she carries to births) and to explore her references and documentation of her training.

Midwives, because they are independent professionals, are able to provide mothers and their families with individual care. They are not bound by the regulations of hospitals or the time limitations of a medical office. In addition, most midwives have borne children and loved the experience. As women and mothers, they are uniquely capable of understanding pregnant women. They have firsthand knowledge of what they teach and do. Because midwives consider themselves your partner in your health care rather than in charge of your health care, you will usually find that you will be comfortable expressing your needs and desires and that they can help you achieve these. Most independent midwives provide prenatal care in their own homes, providing you with a comfortable and informal atmosphere. They will also do at least one prenatal visit at your home prior to the birth.

Because most midwives rely on low-tech diagnostic techniques using their common sense, intuition, and sensitivity, many midwives are uniquely able to detect and avert pregnancy problems without the use of invasive (and expensive) procedures. Because midwives tend to choose their profession out of their deep caring for mothers and babies, they will provide you with excellent continuous care, seeing you from the time you initially contact them through the first months after your baby is born. Unlike other practitioners, most midwives make themselves readily available to their clients by phone for questions and concerns, in addition to being on call by pager for urgent situations. However, because midwives are not recognized as members of the medical profession in most states, nor are they trained to perform certain emergency medical procedures, your midwife is unlikely to be able to continue to provide you with treatment should an emergency arise and transport to the hospital becomes necessary.

In the states where midwives are treated with hostility, your midwife might not be able to accompany you to the hospital, or, if she does, may prefer to accompany you provided you do not refer to her as a midwife. In states where midwifery is legal, or where there are supportive obstetricians willing to serve as a medical liaison to the hospital in case of emergency, a backup physician can be obtained before the birth. It is important that you discuss the issue of an emergency at some point during the pregnancy and decide upon a clear course of action. Most midwives will have clear protocols that they can explain to you.

If you are working with either a direct-entry midwife or a nurse-midwife, she should be able to provide you with the name of an obstetrician if you are not a candidate for a home birth or a birthing center birth, or should medical problems arise during your pregnancy. If you are at risk or have developed problems, you may need to work with an obstetrician, but you may in addition want to work with a midwife as a consultant, as problems of pregnancy and birth can often be reduced. In such cases, a team of health care providers can be ideal.

When choosing a health care practitioner, always ask questions that are important to you and will help you choose the most appropriate practitioner for you.

Here are some questions to ask a midwife you are interviewing:

- What is your training and level of experience?

- What are your midwifery credentials?

- Are you involved in continuing education?

- How do you handle various complications and emergencies?

- What is your medical backup or contingency plan for emergencies?

- What will be your role in an emergency? Will you continue to be with me during the emergency even if I have to go to the hospital?

- What kind of equipment do you carry? Do you know how to use this equipment?

- Do you intend to see me with an assistant or by yourself? What about births?

- Is there a backup care provider should you be ill or otherwise unavailable at any point during the pregnancy or the birth?

- What are your fees and what do they cover? Are any expenses covered by medical insurance? Am I entitled to any reimbursement in the event that I need to transfer out of your practice, for instance, if there is an emergency and a planned home birth becomes unfeasible?

- What are your philosophies about birth?

You must be honest and comfortable with your care providers if they are really to meet your needs. It is of the utmost importance that you work with someone you trust, whether this be a practitioner with an unconventional training or a formally trained physician. If you aren't comfortable, seek another practitioner. This is your pregnancy and your decision to make. Ideally, your mate should feel comfortable with this person as well. The practitioner should respect you as an equal and talk to you with respect, answer your questions directly, and never treat you in a condescending way. If you feel that you are being treated in a way that makes you uncomfortable, find another practitioner with whom you do feel comfortable. In birthing, it is essential that you can be open, both literally and figuratively, and that your confidence in yourself be nurtured and reinforced.

## DO-IT-YOURSELF BIRTHS

A very small number of women are choosing DIY pregnancies and birth, with the philosophy that since birth is completely natural, why have anyone there? In truth, I've been there and done that in the absence of optimal midwifery options in a home-birth hostile environment. While in truth, most births go well and even beautifully (even without a skilled attendant if mom is healthy to begin with), emergencies can arise unexpectedly, which can leave you, your partner, relative, friend, or whomever is supporting you holding the bag, so to speak. This is a heavy emotional burden if things don't turn out well. While excellent self-care and intuitive awareness can guide you through pregnancy and birth safely, joyously, and in optimal health, and a DIY birth can be an empowering experience, you also have to really consider the responsibility and consequences, and still have some emergency contingency plans. It is also important to retain enough humility to ask for help, support, advice, or information at any time you want or need them, and that you be uncompromisingly committed to yours and baby's well-being over ideology.

# Prenatal Visits

Prenatal visits should provide the opportunity for you (and your family) to have personalized and intimate time with someone who is knowledgeable about pregnancy and birth, who can answer your questions and give you information, support, encouragement, and confirmation of the baby's growth and health as well as your own. It is also a time when a basic prenatal examination can indicate if there are any problems developing that require further assessment, treatment, or just watching. Prenatal visits should provide a chance for you and your care provider to get to know each other, developing a comfortable relationship that you can call upon for support during your pregnancy, birth, and transition to motherhood. During these visits, your care provider should also help dad and siblings to feel the baby, listen to the baby's heartbeat, and so on. This helps all members of the family develop a deep prenatal bond with the baby and also lessens the difficulty of introducing a new baby to older siblings. In my experience, children who have been well integrated into prenatal care readily accept their siblings and often participate in their care. A wise practitioner will always honor the primary relationship of the parents and do what she can to foster communication between them, helping the father accept his role as an active participant.

Prenatal care can vary greatly depending upon the type of practitioner you are seeing and her personal philosophy. The setting in which your prenatal visits occur, the regulations to which your practitioner is subjected, and the extent to which you help to shape your own care also matter.

## MIDWIFE VISITS

Midwives almost universally take a woman-centered, biopsychosocial approach to prenatal care. That means they want to know who *you* are, how this pregnancy is affecting your life, and how your life affects your experience of pregnancy and might impact your birth. Personal attention is almost a hallmark of midwife-provided prenatal care. Most midwives spend at least thirty minutes to an hour with their clients per prenatal visit. And note that you are more likely to be referred to as a client than a patient! This depth of relationship is beneficial to a pregnant woman as well as her family. It can raise your sense of comfort, enabling you to relax your inhibitions and discuss personal issues that might affect your health, such as marital stress, herpes outbreaks, or parenting concerns. It can also reduce your anxiety about entering labor. And you are more likely to be willing to discuss intimate physical discomforts and concerns with your midwife that you might be reluctant to discuss with a male practitioner.

The setting for prenatal care is generally the midwife's home, office, or your own home. A more typically casual environment than a medical office, in my opinion, increases your perception that pregnancy is a normal, everyday event—that birth can also occur in a relaxed, comfortable, and nonmedical environment. Your midwife is likely to include you in all procedures, teaching you if you're interested, and encouraging you if you're not, to be an active participant in your prenatal care. Your prenatal care becomes a nonmedical experience, and more of a perfect chance for you to learn about the process of pregnancy, how your body works, and how to optimally prepare for birth and mothering.

Group prenatal care is an exciting and terrific option that some practices offer. It allows you to meet other women due close to when you are, and, in sharing concerns and questions with each other and your midwife, you might find some reassurance and connection—even some support for each other after your babies are born! Of course, make sure you also have some one-on-one visits with your midwife so you can discuss personal and private issues as needed.

## OBSTETRICIAN VISITS

While there are some excellent obstetricians who provide holistic medical care and spend time familiarizing themselves with their patients' needs, most of these office visits will be brief, with the pregnant woman sometimes seeing the doctor for only fifteen minutes or less each time. The advantage of working with an obstetrician is that she or he can provide you with continuity of care in situations ranging from a normal vaginal birth to a complicated cesarean section. Since about half of all obstetricians are men, you may find yourself inhibited in some discussions, even to the point of enduring certain physical discomforts, such as a symptomatic yeast infection, because you are too embarrassed to discuss the vaginal itching and discharge. You may also hesitate to discuss difficulty in your sexual relationship for similar reasons of embarrassment.

When working with most obstetricians, you are not likely to be involved in the medical aspects of your care, such as understanding routine tests and procedures. While some women may prefer not to take this responsibility, I believe that participating in your pregnancy empowers you as a woman. Your care provider should not be more knowledgeable about your body than you are.

# Prenatal Testing

The United States spends more on prenatal testing than any other country in the world, yet we do not rank anywhere near the top twenty countries in terms of optimal outcomes for mother and baby. In fact, we are hovering down at about thirty-fifth in infant mortality![1] U.S. obstetrics practices treat pregnancy as a medical event to be managed and monitored with blood tests, ultrasounds, amniocentesis, and other often unnecessary interventions.

To optimize pregnancy health and the health of our babies, we'd do better with an emphasis on nutritional awareness and other aspects of physical wellness, such as exercise and rest, and on the emotional and psychological health of the mother and the family. There are also many noninvasive, harmless methods of monitoring

---

1. National Research Council and Institute of Medicine, *U.S. Health in International Perspective: Shorter Lives, Poorer Health,* (Washington, DC: The National Academies Press, 2013).

pregnancy progress and maternal and fetal well-being; for example, keeping tabs on blood pressure, and weight, measuring the growth of the uterus abdominally using a tape measure to assess for amount of amniotic fluid and fetal growth, feeling for the baby's position by examining your belly, and listening to the baby's heart rate—even using a fetoscope rather than ultrasound or Doppler. Additional tests can be added as needed for medical reasons rather than simply done routinely or for medico-legal reasons. Fear of litigation should an obstetrician not detect a problem leads practitioners to employ tests, protecting their own professional and personal interests and offsetting legal claims against them.

Standard prenatal lab tests, which usually check blood type and Rh factor, hemoglobin, and an analysis of red and white blood cells, as well as ascertaining whether there is an immunity to rubella (German measles) or toxoplasmosis (contracted from handling infected cat feces and ingesting raw meat, both of which should be avoided by all pregnant women) are reasonable as routine tests as is testing for HIV, Hepatitis B, syphilis, and other sexually transmitted infections if you are at risk.

*When you are pregnant is a perfect time to get information about how your body works.* ❧

More than ever, invasive—and sometimes unreliable—procedures have become routine components of prenatal care. A mere twenty years ago, many tests such as amniocentesis were performed only if problems were suspected or there were significant risk factors. Other tests, such as chorionic villi sampling, were not yet developed. The increase in such tests' availability has led to them becoming entirely routine in the obstetrician's office.

Every obstetric test has advantages and disadvantages. For example, knowing that she will give birth to a child with Down syndrome, as revealed by an amniocentesis, may enable a woman and her partner to prepare for this, emotionally, psychologically, and materially, and find resources, organizations, and special supplies that they will need for caring for their child. Or if they choose to abort the child, they will avoid the stress that they perceive will accompany both raising a Down syndrome child and the stress the child might experience in a society that is often discriminatory. However, the amniocentesis procedure can also cause damage to an otherwise perfectly healthy fetus or even cause the miscarriage of a normal baby. It is up to each woman to become educated about the risks and benefits of the tests available to her prenatally and to develop the confidence to agree to tests that she does want done and to refuse the rest. It is essential that we examine our routine reliance on such equipment and tests as the Doppler and diagnostic ultrasound, alpha-fetoprotein, chorionic villi sampling, and amniocentesis during pregnancy. In addition to their potential harm to the baby—about which much is still unknown—these tests externalize the mother's authority and body wisdom, keeping her distanced from the trust she might otherwise learn to develop in herself. This is not to say that testing is always unnecessary; it can be a great relief to a concerned mother to know that her baby appears to be healthy and growing well; it can also provide invaluable life-saving information when a problem is suspected.

Following are explanations of the purpose, procedure, risks, and benefits of several of the more common prenatal tests that might be considered invasive. I use the term *invasive* to mean that these tests require penetrating the body, either directly or by sound waves, or that they have the potential for harmful effects. Prenatal testing is an important issue in prenatal care, particularly if you are working with a medical practitioner, and I therefore encourage you to read *Pursuing the Birth Machine* by Marsden Wagner, The *Encyclopedia of Childbearing* by Barbara Katz-Rothman, *Obstetric Myths versus Research Realities* by Henci Goer, and *Immaculate Deception* by Suzanne Arms (see Bibliography, page 271).

*It is up to each woman to become educated about the risks and benefits of the tests available to her prenatally, and to develop the confidence to agree to tests that she does want done, and to refuse the rest.*

## DOPPLER ULTRASOUND

The Doppler is an electronic device used routinely at a prenatal examination by both doctors and nurse-midwives, and occasionally by midwives, to hear the fetal heartbeat. It can detect the fetal heartbeat as early as eight weeks into the pregnancy. The Doppler works by directing a continuous sound wave at the baby, which is then received by the amplification device and makes the heartbeat audible to those in the room. Many women enjoy hearing their baby's heartbeat amplified but do not question the safety of the Doppler. In fact, the Doppler has not been conclusively proven safe for use in pregnancy; not enough long-term evidence is available. Nor has the Doppler been proven more effective or accurate in assessing fetal heart tones than the completely benign use of the fetoscope, a fetal stethoscope. One minute of exposure to Doppler has been estimated as equivalent to thirty-five minutes of imaging ultrasound exposure. The Doppler is very useful for hearing the fetal heartbeat when it is difficult to hear it manually. You may want to request that your care provider use the fetoscope in place of routine use of the Doppler, reserving its use for medical necessity, such as when the safety of the fetus is of concern and the heartbeat is inaudible with a fetoscope (for example, in the event of threatened miscarriage or lack of normal fetal movement).

## DIAGNOSTIC ULTRASOUND (ULTRASONOGRAPHY, SONOGRAPHY)

Imaging ultrasound employs a similar technology to the Doppler ultrasound but produces a screen image of the fetus and the placenta, which can be evaluated diagnostically. It is used routinely—most pregnant American women can expect to have at least one, and frequently several, ultrasounds. It too has not been proven safe for use in pregnancy.

While pregnant women find it exciting or reassuring to see a picture of their baby, imaging ultrasound is more appropriately reserved for use when there are medical indications such as suspected fetal demise, suspected placenta previa, a significant size/dates discrepancy, and determination of fetal position if it is difficult to determine it with palpation alone. If you do require an ultrasound, you can request that it be done by a technician with a lot of experience in order to reduce the amount of time that you are exposed and to get the most accurate reading.

## PRENATAL SCREENING

Alpha-fetoprotein (AFP) is a chemical produced by your baby's liver, minute quantities of which appear in your bloodstream. The level of AFP rises progressively throughout pregnancy. Maternal blood levels are assessed for the amount of AFP and other chemicals present; an abnormally low or high level may indicate the presence of fetal anomalies. This test may be performed routinely without your knowledge at the time of your initial prenatal lab screening. MSAFP is not a harmful test; however, it has a high rate of false positives. When a woman is determined to have abnormal AFP levels, she is then referred for further testing, usually an amniocentesis. Frequently, then, the woman will be anxious until the amniocentesis is performed. She will then be exposed to tests with higher risks for the mother and baby. The optimal time to have the MSAFP test performed is between fifteen and eighteen weeks' gestation, as the test is thought to be the most accurate when done during this time. When a fetus is determined without a doubt to have anomalies, the hard choice then arises as to whether to keep the pregnancy or abort.

## AMNIOCENTESIS

To perform an amniocentesis, a doctor inserts a long, sterile needle through your abdominal and uterine walls into the amniotic fluid. This test is done with an ultrasound in order to view the fetus and placenta. The amniotic fluid that is collected contains fetal cells that will provide information on fetal well-being and can indicate whether the fetus has certain birth defects (such as Down syndrome), hemolytic anemia (destruction of the red blood cells that occurs from Rh disease), and many diseases, including cystic fibrosis as well as carbohydrate, fat, and amino acid metabolic disorders. It can be used to determine lung maturity when a premature labor is occurring or if a preterm cesarean section is necessary.

*We have become so highly acculturated to accepting birth as a technological and medical event that we must unlearn cultural conditioning.*

Risks include puncturing the umbilical cord, placenta, or uterus, or causing infection or miscarriage. In addition, if an insufficient amount of fluid is collected, or if the culture of the fetal cells doesn't grow, the test will need to repeated.

If the baby is determined to have a disorder, you must then choose whether to keep the baby or abort. Amniocentesis cannot screen for all possible fetal disorders, and it can potentially damage a normal fetus. You must weigh the risks and benefits of having this test done, especially if you plan to keep the baby no matter what the problem is.

## CHORIONIC VILLI SAMPLING (CVS)

To perform this test (at between nine and eleven weeks' gestation), tissues are removed from what will develop into the placenta. The tissue is obtained by going through either the abdomen or cervix, and using an instrument to remove the tissue while directly looking at the area. This test can check for chromosomal abnormalities, but cannot detect all of the problems that can be picked up by amniocentesis.

Risks of this test include damaging the embryo (damage can be as severe as the loss of a limb), damage to the cervix and uterus, infection, hemorrhage, and miscarriage. This test should not be done in the presence of a vaginal infection, Rh sensitization, or multiple gestation. I seriously suspect other potential problems we've not yet discovered, as disrupting the placenta is a significant interruption of what nature intended.

As with other diagnostic tests, you must evaluate the risk-to-benefit ratio. If you plan to abort the baby if there is a problem, CVS can provide you with quick and early diagnosis. (Results are usually available in twenty-four hours.) If you plan to keep the baby if there is a problem, you must keep in mind that an otherwise healthy baby can suffer severe damage as a result of this procedure.

# Childbirth Education Classes

Our bodies know how to birth. However, we have become so highly acculturated to accepting birth as a technological and medical event that natural birth and women-empowerment-oriented childbirth classes can actually be a tool for helping us to *unlearn* the cultural conditioning that can undermine our efforts to birth naturally. Also, few of us have older women in our lives who can guide and advise us about natural pregnancy and birth—a childbirth educator who herself has children can fill this gap wonderfully. Finally, childbirth classes can connect us with other couples going through what we're going through, and this can provide not only support but a reminder that everything you're going through is pretty normal for pregnancy! For example, many couples experience sexual tension during pregnancy (one partner may want more physical intimacy than the other) or confusion and anger over unmet expectations (pregnant women may want their mates to be more involved in touching the baby or buying baby clothes than the partner cares to be). Talking about it as a group and realizing that you aren't the only ones can help you laugh about it and get more relaxed. Many pregnant women experience similar physical and emotional challenges, and many men feel unsure in their new role.

Childbirth education classes provide a forum for parents to explore such issues under the guidance of a childbirth educator, usually a woman (or a couple) who has knowledge about pregnancy and birth through both study and personal experience. While midwives can provide excellent prenatal education that can often substitute for prenatal classes, the opportunity to share and learn with other couples is very valuable, particularly for first-time parents. In an obstetrician's office, rarely is there time allocated for prenatal education. Classes in this case are also necessary if you are to have any understanding of the birth process or hospital procedures and protocols.

There are numerous childbirth education organizations offering their own philosophies, material, and educational styles. Classes offered in hospitals are nearly always geared toward a hospital birth. While *natural childbirth* might be a phrase that regularly pops up in the discussion, you are also likely to receive complete information on the drugs of choice for pain relief, full preparation for a cesarean section, and minimal information that would truly support you in achieving either a natural pregnancy or birth. If a truly positive and natural experience is your goal, you will want to seek a childbirth teacher who is well versed in positive, natural birth and who orients classes toward home birth or home and hospital birth. Whether you are planning a home or hospital birth, it is imperative that the classes educate you about medical procedures commonly used during birth so that you can discriminate between necessary procedures and hospital policies, protocols that might expose you to unnecessary testing, and intervention that the hospital requires in order to reduce its insurance liabilities. It is your right to exercise authority over your own body.

Ideally, classes should begin in early pregnancy in order to address the needs of pregnant mothers, couples, and families. For example, there should be discussion of nutrition and common discomforts during each trimester, discussion of emotional issues that are likely to arise, and preparation for the experience of pregnancy and parenting, of which birth is just a part (albeit a very profound part). Classes that encourage you to focus mainly on breathing techniques will distract you from finding your own strength, and in a subtle way promote a fear of birth. Such classes may stress the necessity of avoiding the pain or intensity of labor. You will know what to do. A good class will help you identify your inner resources for birth and prepare you for parenting and breastfeeding. A good class will help you find confidence in your abilities, while welcoming the intensity of birth and parenting.

In the resources section, you will find organizations that offer childbirth education services with trained teachers around the United States, Canada, and Europe. Midwives often offer classes to their clients and so do hospitals. If not, they can recommend childbirth educators in your area.

The Internet is an incredibly rich source of pregnancy, birth, and mommy information—but remember, not every expert is really an expert and not all information is reliable!

# CHAPTER 5

# What to Eat When You're Pregnant

>>>><<<<

*I'm sorry to tell you this*, but we've got a big problem, *a serious and growing problem.* Our children are in danger.

This generation of children—our children and grandchildren—are the first in history to have an anticipated life expectancy *shorter* than that of its parents. Along with this, rates of autism have been escalating, with an estimated one in sixty-eight children on the spectrum according to the CDC.[1] Approximately 11 percent of children aged 4 to 17 (6.4 million) have been diagnosed with ADHD as of 2011, according to the *Journal of the American Academy of Child and Adolescent Psychiatry*.[2] Type 2 diabetes, which just a couple of decades ago was a disease of adults, has now skyrocketed in tweens and teens according to studies published by the American Medical Association.[3]

What's the good news? The solution is simple, and it's right at the end of our forks! Feed our kids right, from the start, ideally *before* and certainly during pregnancy.

Nutrition is the cornerstone of a healthy pregnancy. It is also the foundation of lifelong health and longevity for our kids.

---

1. CDC, "Prevalence of Autism Spectrum Disorder Among Children Aged 8 Years—Autism and Developmental Disabilities Monitoring Network," *MMWR* 2014; 63 (No. SS 2): 1-21.

2. Stephen J. Blumburg et al., "Trends in the Parent-Report of Health Care Provider-Diagnosed and Medicated Attention-Deficit/Hyperactivity Disorder: United States, 2003–2011," *Journal of the American Academy of Child & Adolescent Psychiatry*, 53, no. 1 (January 2014): 34-46.e2.

3. Dana Dabelea et al., "Prevalence of Type 1 and Type 2 Diabetes Among Children and Adolescents From 2001 to 2009," *JAMA*, 2014;311(17):1778-1786, doi:10.1001/jama.2014.3201.

Yet nutrition counseling remains one of the most underemphasized aspects of conventional prenatal care. Why? Its role in optimal health, while well established, is undervalued—practically ignored by medicine. It is not something pharmaceutical companies can sell. It is not a surgical intervention that makes big bucks for hospitals. In fact, educating patients about nutrition is time and labor intensive. Most docs think it doesn't pay. Yet ignoring it comes with high costs to individual patients, to society, and to you and me and our kids! We spend more on chronic disease in one year in the United States than the combined gross national product of several large European countries! Yet these diseases are largely preventable with nutrition—starting even before we are pregnant.

Obesity, diabetes, cancer, allergies, asthma, ADD/ADHD, and autism are just a few examples of conditions that are on the rise and are associated with food and nutrition. It appears that prenatal vulnerability stems from possible "programming," whereby adaptations made by the fetus at a critical or sensitive developmental period in intrauterine life, has permanent effects on structure, physiology, and metabolism.

It is believed that cardiovascular disease, for example, may be a consequence of fetal adaptations in insulin release and cholesterol metabolism to undernutrition that are beneficial for short-term survival, but have long-term consequences—particularly creating tissue responsiveness to insulin similar to insulin resistance. Low birth weight (independent of prematurity) due to intrauterine undernutrition is associated with later development of hypertension, diabetes, elevated serum cholesterol and fibrinogen concentrations, and polycystic ovary syndrome, which is actually a metabolic disease similar to insulin resistance and with all of the same risk factors as DM2. It is well documented that adult diseases related to poor prenatal nutrition transcend social groups, maternal smoking, alcohol intake, and mom having diabetes.

## Optimal Nutrition

Optimal nutrition is a way of loving and caring for ourselves and our babies that maximizes our fullest potential. It is also the nurturing stuff that life is made of! Who doesn't feel better when a close relative or friend serves us a bowl of warm soup and we feel that we are being fed much more than the food itself.

Most health care providers are painfully ignorant about healthy food and nutrition. What I share with you here is a combination of conventional knowledge combined with what *should* be taught about nutrition, but isn't: preventative nutritional strategies for maintaining optimal pregnancy health and growing really healthy babies.

Optimal pregnancy health not only helps to ensure that your baby is healthy, intelligent, and resistant to infections, but will ensure that you are healthy during the pregnancy and birth. So many women consider the common "complaints" of pregnancy to be normal. But persistent constipation, headaches, leg cramps, and exhaustion can be prevented or relieved with good nutrition—in fact many are a sign of inadequate or improper nutrition! Eating well lays a foundation of health that can support you when you are breastfeeding during the precious first few years of your child's life. It will also help you meet the demands every parent of young children must face. A well-nourished person is better able to cope with stress than one who is inadequately nourished.

So what do you need to know for optimal pregnancy nutrition?

## Getting Started

The first step you can take toward optimal nutrition is simply to make the commitment to make everything you eat count toward health. You and your baby deserve it! Planning ahead for shopping and meal prep with menus that you organize perhaps once a week can really help if you hate cooking, are really busy with other kids and social activities, and/or have a job outside the home that interferes with eating well. A few good cookbooks or foodie websites with recipes can make a world of difference in food planning and can keep you from getting bored with the same old same old. There will be days when you just don't feel like cooking—but you still need to eat well. Have great snacks and quick healthy packaged foods on hand. With stores like Whole Foods and Trader Joe's, there is no shortage of options. Without some advance planning meals are likely to be missed or skimped on. Significant others? Get involved with the meal planning, prep, and creation—it's your baby's future, too!

*For each of us as women, there is a deep place within, where hidden and growing our true spirit rises. . . . Within these deep places, each one holds an incredible reserve of creativity and power, of unexamined and unrecorded emotion and feeling.*

—AUDRE LORDE

## MINDFUL EATING

Eating optimally starts with eating mindfully. Excellent nutrition is more than just taking in a certain number of recommended daily allowances: it is also an awareness of how we prepare, eat, and digest our food; of how we feel about our bodies as well as our emotional, mental, and spiritual selves; of what chemicals are in the foods we eat and how these affect not only our own health, but also our baby's health and the health of our environment. Mindful eating means taking a minute before making a food choice to make sure you're making an optimally healthy choice and that you're eating because you're hungry—not out of boredom, fatigue, stress, sadness, or other nonhunger reasons. In other words, think before you eat.

# We Bring Home More than the Bacon: Hidden Dangers in Our Foods

In addition to what we are eating, we have to think about what's in what we're eating—and what packaging our foods come in. In truth, it's kind of a lot of work. The evidence is clear—by the time they are born, our babies are already contaminated with over three hundred chemicals measurable in their umbilical cord blood. These chemicals can cause birth defects, diabetes, cancer, and a host of other problems. And we haven't even begun to scientifically understand what the chemicals do in combination in our bodies! There are toxic residues from agricultural contaminants such as pesticides on produce and antibiotics fed to animals; even food packaging and cooking supplies (BPA in plastic bottles, teflon and PFOA [perfluorooctanoic acid] from nonstick pans, for example) that we're exposed to during pregnancy have profound and potentially lifelong negative implications for our children's health.

### Supporting the Community

Low income women and women of color have significantly higher rates of mortality, morbidity, and having babies with congenital problems. It is essential that our communities find ways to support those women who are at greater risk, such as providing free prenatal classes, promoting social services that provide prenatal care, and starting community gardens to provide seasonal fresh vegetables to pregnant women.

We can minimize the chemical "body burden" our kids will experience by following some simple rules:

- Eat organic whenever possible or at least avoid the "dirty dozen," the list put out by the nonprofit Environmental Working Group of the most contaminated foods. The list is updated annually and can be found at www.ewg.org/foodnews/index.php. If you need to purchase nonorganic, choose from the "Clean 15," also found at the EWG website.

- Avoid plastic wrap and storage containers.

- Eat only organic, grass-fed, antibiotic-free meats and dairy.

- Avoid high-mercury fish including mackerel (king), marlin, orange roughy, shark, swordfish, tilefish, and tuna (bigeye, ahi).

- Eat fish no more than twice weekly, and avoid farm-raised fish, which is high in PCBs (polychlorinated biphenyls).

- Avoid exposure to household, industrial, and agricultural chemicals, and even many cosmetics, which can contain lead, mercury, and other toxic chemicals!

# What Should You Eat?

Eat a rainbow. No, I'm not kidding, and I'm not talking about Skittles, either! Eat a wide variety of brightly colored vegetable and fruits in as close to a natural form as possible. Eat low-mercury fish, chicken, and red meat—or a healthy vegetarian diet replete with grains and beans. Eat nuts, seeds, and good quality oils. If you tolerate it, eat organic dairy. Drink water and gentle herbal teas as your beverages. Voilà: A healthy diet!

So many of us worry about whether we're getting enough to meet our growing baby's nutritional needs. Believe it or not, you don't need that much more when you're pregnant than when you're not. Actually, if you eat a generally healthy diet and increase your intake by about 300 calories per day (the calorie equivalent, to help you get the picture, of a glass of milk and half a sandwich—though you don't have to drink milk to be healthy in pregnancy)—you'll actually be getting most of what you need for a healthy pregnancy. Add to that about 400 micrograms of folic acid or folate (up to 1 gram if you have something called an MTHFR polymorphism—ask you're midwife or obstetrician about this), about 18 grams of iron (which you can get from food), and a bit of calcium, and you're just about there. So you can see that there's very little to worry about if you're on a healthy, whole foods diet!

# The Nutrients

Here are some general guidelines to the foods and servings you need to eat daily:

- **Protein:** This should comprise 20 percent of a normal pregnancy diet. The recommended daily allowance (RDA) in pregnancy is 60 grams (about four servings), which most Americans meet, though vegetarians and vegans may need to pay extra attention to get enough.

- **Carbohydrates:** These should comprise 50 percent during pregnancy and can come from *whole* grains and vegetables. That's about four to six servings.

- **Vitamin C foods:** Have two servings.

- **Calcium foods:** Have four servings.

- **Green leafy vegetables and yellow fruits and vegetables:** Have three servings.

- **Other veggies and fruits:** Have one to two servings,

- **Iron-rich foods:** Have some daily.

- **Good-quality high-fat foods:** Have two servings.

- **Salt:** Can be used daily, in moderation, to taste.

- **Fluids:** Have at least six to eight glasses a day.

- **Fiber:** If you're getting all of the above, you should be getting enough.

- Note that all of these requirements increase when you are carrying two or more babies.

Remember, this is an ideal that you should try to achieve as closely as possible. You will have better days and skimpier days, depending on how you feel and what is going on in your life. I also suggest that you pay attention to how you feel when you eat or miss a meal, or compare the feeling of when you eat a healthy meal to when you eat a sweet snack or junk food (which I hope you'll generally avoid). In time, your body will come to crave the healthy meals over the empty foods.

Foods eaten during pregnancy should be highly "nutrient dense"—that is, should contain a high amount of protein, vitamins, and minerals per 100 calories (also called kcal for kilocalorie) of food . This means that you should avoid "empty calories," which usually come in the form of junk food—including natural food junk food substitutes!

How do you get these nutrients? Foods are always the best sources of nutrition—and major food sources of these nutrients are described below. A prenatal vitamin can provide a little extra insurance—especially when you have days when you just don't eat as well—which happens now and then in pregnancy—and a good prenatal vitamin also compensates for the nutrients missing from our soil. What if prenatal vitamins nauseate you? Talk with an integrative doctor about taking betaine HCL to help you tolerate your vitamin better, take your vitamin with or after food, don't take it early in the morning or before bed, and if pills turn your stomach, find a food-based good-quality liquid prenatal vitamin.

Following are descriptions of the common essential nutrients, along with their functions and the sources from which you can obtain them.

## PROTEIN

Protein is one of the most abundant substances in the body, second only to water. It provides the structural framework upon which all body tissues depend for healthy growth. Bones, muscles, skin, blood, hair, nails, organs, and connective tissue are all made from proteins. The baby's hormones, growth, metabolism, and sexual development are made possible with protein. Protein is necessary for basic chemical reactions, including the maintenance of fluid and pH balance. Protein encourages and contributes to the formation of antibodies necessary for fighting infection. A diet with an emphasis on good quality protein and complex carbohydrates is best for keeping blood sugar levels—and our energy—steady.

Protein provides the raw material for making a baby, placenta, and strong uterus. It contributes to the formation of breast milk and is essential for healthy blood clotting. There are about twenty-two amino acids—the structural components of protein and the end products of protein digestion—needed by the body. All but eight of these can be produced in the body or converted into another kind should a shortage of any occur. The eight that must be obtained from your diet are called *essential amino acids*. These eight amino acids are available in many foods in varying proportions. However, for the protein to be used optimally by the body, they need to be present in specific amounts. Foods in which the amino acids are always present in these specific quantities are known as *complete proteins*. These include such foods as meats, dairy products, and soybean products. When eating meat as a protein source, organic is preferable. Though it may be slightly more expensive than inorganic meat, avoiding the many chemical contaminants found in meat (antibiotics, growth hormones, and other chemicals given to animals during their growth) is preferable for the health of both the mother and the baby. Foods such as grains, seeds, nuts, and legumes are known as *incomplete proteins* as they are either missing or low in specific amino acids. When eaten in various combinations, grains and legumes form complete proteins that are highly nutritious and assimilable by the body. Vegetables also contain usable proteins but in smaller amounts than the foods already mentioned. (See below for a discussion of protein combining.)

Protein is not well stored in the body, and a continual supply is necessary for the healthy functioning of all of our cells. Protein deficiency may manifest itself in abnormal growth and development, loss of muscle tone, lack of vigor and stamina, mental depression, increased susceptibility to infection, poor wound healing, and slow recovery from illness. Protein loss occurs through stresses such as injury and illness. During such times, extra protein is required to replace or repair tissues.

Childbearing, with the increased size and amount of the mother's tissues, the baby's needs, labor, birth, postpartum healing, and lactation, requires a great increase in protein consumption. While protein requirements are influenced by a woman's size, nutritional status, and activity levels, it is generally thought that 75 to 100 grams of protein daily will fulfill the protein requirement for pregnancy. Eating at least four servings per day of protein-rich foods as part of meals, with complementary high-protein snacks (such as yogurt, cheese and crackers, or hummus dip) daily will provide you with adequate protein. I personally have found that the lower end of this range is optimal, the upper end producing very large babies and difficult digestion. Inadequate protein intake during pregnancy is associated with eclampsia.

## CARBOHYDRATES

Carbohydrates are the main source of energy for all body functions, including digestion and assimilation of food and all muscular activity. Carbohydrates provide immediately available energy for producing heat in the body. Broken down into glucose, carbohydrates provide fuel for the brain, nervous system, and muscle tissues; in the form of glycogen, carbohydrates can be stored by the liver and muscles. Carbohydrates, when available in excess, can also be stored throughout the body in the form of fat and used as reserve energy when needed. (The utilization of fat results in weight loss.)

Carbohydrates are needed in the largest quantity of all the nutrients required by the body. They make up the bulk of our diet. They are available in three main forms: simple sugars, starches (complex carbohydrates), and cellulose (the indigestible parts of fruits and vegetables that provide us with the fiber needed for healthy bowel functioning).

Simple sugars can be found in both refined foods (sugar, candy, soft drinks, chocolate, and so on) and unrefined foods (honey, maple syrup, and other natural sweeteners as well as fruits). In these forms, they are almost immediately digested, quickly raising blood sugar levels and eliminating feelings of hunger. It is important to realize that the feeling of hunger, although triggered somewhat by falling blood sugar levels, is more than a signal to put more sugar in the body. It is also a call for vital nutrients. Both refined and unrefined sugars have the ability to satisfy hunger with quick fuel. This can lead us to forgo eating nutritious foods that will provide us with longer-lasting energy. This is true for fruits as well, though they do provide essential vitamins and minerals. Since excess carbohydrates are stored in the body as fat, you can actually become overweight at the same time you are becoming malnourished. Simple sugars are short-lived in the bloodstream, leaving us with sudden feelings of fatigue, depression, irritability, headache, and the need for another boost of energy. Persistent overconsumption of simple sugars can also lead to an overly large baby and maternal diabetes (with complications for both mom and baby).

*The powerful world of pregnancy holds the joys and the awe of creating a whole new person who will be part of your life, indefinitely.*

—JOY GARDNER

Starches are complex chains of sugar units. When carbohydrates are eaten in this form, the sugar units are separated and digested slowly, thus taking longer to reach the bloodstream and satiate hunger. This slow digestion allows the body adequate time to absorb the range of nutrients in these unprocessed starchy foods. With complex carbohydrates, blood sugar levels remain steady for a longer time than with simple sugars, so hunger is sated for a considerably greater length of time.

If carbohydrate intake is insufficient, the body will use protein and fat for energy. This leads to a harmful chemical residue in the body known as *ketones*, which if present consistently or in high amounts can be dangerous for both the mother and the baby. It is therefore essential that pregnant mothers base their diets around complex carbohydrates as their source of energy (four to six servings daily), getting these from whole grains (brown rice, whole wheat, millet, oats, rye, barley, amaranth, and so on), seeds, and a variety of starchy vegetables such as squashes and beets. If you are at risk for or have gestational diabetes, you will want to minimize your carbohydrate intake from grains and sweet, starchy vegetables.

## FATS

Fats, or lipids, are the most concentrated form of energy in the diet, providing twice as many calories per gram as carbohydrates and protein. Fats act as carriers of the fat-soluble vitamins—A, D, E, and K. By aiding in the absorption of vitamin D, fats make calcium available to body tissues. Also, fats are important in converting carotene to vitamin A. Fat deposits surround, hold in place, and protect major organs. A layer of body fat helps the body deal with temperature changes in a room or outdoors and preserves body heat. There are three essential fatty acids (substances that give fats their different properties such as melting point, flavor, and texture). They are synthesized by the body if one of them, linoleic acid, is present in the diet. These unsaturated fatty acids are necessary for healthy blood, arteries, nerves, skin, and other tissues. They aid in the digestion of cholesterol.

Cholesterol is a fat-related substance and is needed to form sex and adrenal hormones, vitamin D, healthy blood, skin, the nervous system, brain and liver tissue, and the bile that is necessary for the digestion of fats.

Although rare, a deficiency of fats will lead to a deficiency of fat-soluble vitamins and related disorders. Excessive intake of fats could also lead to digestive and other health problems. An acceptable intake is one tablespoon (Tb) of fat daily in the form of a pure vegetable oil (unrefined, cold-pressed oil), as well as foods rich in this nutrient. Significant sources of fats are nuts, seeds, vegetable oils, butter, margarine, dairy products, and fats in meat. Salmon, sardines, and herring are excellent sources of essential fatty acids and can be eaten a couple of times a week. Essential fatty acids are also found in the oils derived from evening primrose, walnuts, black currants, flaxseeds, and borage. Raw walnut oil or flaxseed oil can be added to salads and other dishes after cooking, or a supplement of 1,500 milligrams of any of these oils, with the exception of walnut oil (do not exceed this dosage unless there is a specific reason for doing so), can be taken daily throughout pregnancy to ensure adequate intake.

## VITAMINS

### Vitamin A

Vitamin A is most noted for its role in preventing and fighting infections. It promotes healthy skin and mucous membranes, strong bones, rich blood, and keen eyesight. Proper digestion of proteins requires the presence of vitamin A. Requirements may vary greatly from person to person, and both deficiency and excess of this vitamin can be harmful. Therefore, it is important to eat foods rich in vitamin A, but to avoid supplementation of this individual vitamin during pregnancy (other than what is in your prenatal vitamin, if you are taking one).

Acute vitamin A poisoning can be recognized by nausea, vomiting, dry skin, diarrhea, hair loss, sore lips, and flaky, itchy skin. This usually only occurs as a result of excessive supplementation and, unless caused by chronic excess, will disappear soon after the vitamin supplement is withdrawn. In early pregnancy, however, excessive supplementation can result in permanent fetal malformations.

Symptoms of vitamin A deficiency include frequent colds and respiratory problems, sinus trouble, rough skin, acne, dandruff, and night blindness.

Vitamin A is destroyed by light, staleness, drying of foods, and chemical fertilizers. It is leached out of the body by ingesting mineral oil. The body accepts vitamin A more easily in foods that are cooked, mashed, or puréed.

Rich sources of this vitamin include yellow and orange fruits, yellow vegetables, dark green vegetables, orange vegetables such as carrots and sweet potatoes, dairy products, eggs (especially the yolk), and liver.

Herbal sources include alfalfa, watercress, nettle, red raspberry leaves, dandelion, comfrey, nori, yellow dock, and lamb's quarters.

### Vitamin B-complex

The B-complex vitamins are grouped because they have similar functions and tend to occur together in nature. For this reason, a deficiency of a single B vitamin is less likely than a general B vitamin deficiency. B vitamins are essential for a healthy nervous system as well as for the metabolism of carbohydrates, fats, and proteins. They also help maintain muscle tone in the gastrointestinal tract and health of the skin, hair, eyes, mouth, and liver. Since they are water-soluble vitamins, they are not stored in the body and must be ingested through the diet on a regular basis. Some of the B vitamins are produced naturally in healthy intestines.

There are quite a few B-complex vitamins. The following are considered especially important for health during pregnancy.

$B_1$ (thiamin) is necessary for children's consistent growth, a healthy nervous system, and good muscle tone in the stomach, intestines, and heart. $B_1$ aids in the conversion of glucose into energy and helps stabilize the appetite and blood sugar by the assimilation of starches and sugars. Signs of deficiency include constipation, loss of appetite, digestive problems, fatigue, apathy, uncertainty of memory, and nervousness. $B_1$ is stored in the body only in very small amounts, so daily intake is necessary. Found in the outer layers of grains, it is usually lost in the refining process. It is destroyed by heat, oxidation, and alkaline substances such as baking soda.

Food sources include whole grains (especially wheat germ), nuts and seeds, legumes, potatoes, peas, nutritional yeast, bananas, and avocados. Herbal sources include dandelion, alfalfa, red clover, red raspberry leaves, nori, kelp, catnip, and watercress.

**B2 (riboflavin)** is necessary for the assimilation and digestion of carbohydrates, fats, and proteins. It aids in cell respiration. Maintenance of healthy skin, nails, hair, and good vision depends on vitamin B2. Signs of deficiency in B2 include digestive troubles, skin and eye problems, cracking at the corners of the mouth, hair loss, poor lactation, sluggishness, retarded growth, dizziness, trembling, urinary difficulty, vaginal itching, and bloating of the body.

This nutrient is found in nutritional yeast, whole grains (especially wheat), dried beans and peas, seeds (especially sunflower), leafy green vegetables, cottage cheese, milk, and organ meats. Herbal sources include rose hips, dandelion, dulse, kelp, and fenugreek.

**B6 (pyridoxine)** is required for a healthy nervous system and utilization of carbohydrates, fats, and proteins. It must be present for the production of antibodies and red blood cells. It helps regulate body fluids and aids in healthy muscle formation and functioning. It is associated with hormonal balance and, because of its importance in digestion and healthy muscles, deficiency is often associated with nausea and leg cramps in pregnancy. Depression may also be caused by a B6 deficiency. B6 is destroyed by heat and ultraviolet light.

Rich food sources include brown rice, wheat bran and germ, blackstrap molasses, nutritional yeast, bananas, salmon, and organ meats.

**B12** is needed for healthy nerve tissue, fetal brain development, the production of genetic material, proper cell division, and the metabolism of many nutrients. Because plants do not require B12 for their growth, plant foods—unless they are fortified or have been fermented (encouraging the growth of bacteria that contain and help our bodies to synthesize B12)—rarely contain this vitamin. Therefore, those on strictly vegan diets, containing absolutely no animal products, should consider using vitamin B12.

Foods that do contain B12 include dairy products (with the exception of butter) and meats. Vegetarian sources include tempeh, miso, and B12-fortified nutritional yeast. However, tempeh and miso contain variable and, according to some, unreliable amounts of B12. Because our bodies need only small amounts of B12, the addition of a small daily amount of dairy or other animal products to the diet will supply enough, as will a prenatal vitamin. Maintaining healthy intestinal flora with yogurt will also help with intrinsic B12 production.

That our bodies store B12 for years is in some ways an advantage but could also prevent deficiency signs from showing up for five or six years. Signs of B12 deficiency include a glossy sore tongue, indigestion, abdominal pains, and diarrhea or constipation. Left untreated, serious mental and nervous problems may develop, and eventually death may occur. *Megaloblastic* and *pernicious anemia* are terms used to describe deficiencies associated with vitamin B12.

**Folic acid** is a water-soluble member of the B-complex group. It's now been about fifteen years since the United States introduced the fortification of grains—primarily wheat and rice—with folic acid to reduce the incidence of neural tube defects. This has largely been a successful effort, with a 25 percent reduction in rates. This singular step was a broadscale acknowledgment that nutritional health before pregnancy can have a significant impact on pregnancy outcome. The U.S. Public Health Service recommends that women of childbearing age obtain 400 micrograms (0.4 milligrams) of folate or folic acid each day.

Folic acid provides these benefits:

- Reduces baby's risk of neural tube birth defects such as spina bifida if taken at least one month prior to conception and though the fourth week of pregnancy.

- Protects against congenital heart defects, cleft lips, limb defects, and urinary tract anomalies.

- Reduces the risk of preterm delivery, low birth weight, and fetal growth restriction.

- Prevents homocysteinemia, a condition that increases the risk of spontaneous abortion, placental abruption, and preeclampsia (women with low folic acid *prior* to pregnancy are already at great risk, which is alleviated by folic acid supplementation).

- May actually protect the fetus from disease when the mother is ill, taking medications, or smoking during pregnancy.

- Reduces the risk of insulin resistance and adult DM2.

- Reduces the risk of autistic spectrum disorders.

Folic acid is needed in much greater amounts during pregnancy, acting as a safeguard against anemia, miscarriage, premature birth, and birth defects. It is available in green leafy vegetables, wheat germ, nutritional yeast, eggs, whole grains, lentils, nuts, milk, and liver. As it is lost in the cooking process, care must be taken to eat raw leafy green vegetables daily and to regularly include several of these other sources in your diet. Women should supplement with at least 400 micrograms of folic acid daily, but if you have a change in your MTFHR gene, you may need between 1 and 4 grams daily of active folate (methylfolate), so speak with your midwife or doctor about this, ideally before you become pregnant, or as early on as possible in pregnancy. Eating plenty of fresh dark leafy greens daily is also a great way to get folate into your diet, but is not always enough to forego a supplement, so supplementation is still advisable.

### Vitamin C (Ascorbic Acid)

Vitamin C is essential for the production of collagen, a protein needed for forming connective tissue in bones, ligaments, and skin, as well as in the healing of wounds and burns. It is needed to produce a healthy placenta, capillaries, and cell walls, and helps to prevent varicosities and hemorrhage. Vitamin C greatly aids in the assimilation of other nutrients, such as folic acid, iron, vitamins A and E, and certain amino acids. It is very helpful in preventing and healing infections and is quickly used up during stressful times. During pregnancy, the daily dosage should not exceed 2,000 milligrams, as it can lead to miscarriage in early pregnancy, and can cause a vitamin C dependency in the baby, which can lead to scurvy in the newborn.

Found in most fresh fruits and vegetables, vitamin C is destroyed by heat, air, and light, and is also lost in cooking water. At least two servings of vitamin C–rich foods should be eaten each day. Excellent sources include green leafy vegetables such as raw or lightly cooked kale and collard greens, strawberries, peppers, citrus fruits, cantaloupe, alfalfa sprouts, and tomatoes.

Herbal sources include rose hips, watercress, dandelion greens, red clover, burdock, nettle, and alfalfa.

### Vitamin D

Vitamin D, really more of a large group of hormones than a vitamin, is traditionally grouped with the fat-soluble vitamins. It is mainly available through exposure to sunlight and ingestion of fatty fish and fish liver oils, with smaller amounts to be found in butter, milk from grazed cows, and egg yolks. Fortified commercial milk is rich in a synthetic form of vitamin D. Many women are deficient and benefit from 1,000 international units (IU) of vitamin D₃ supplementation daily. Adequate vitamin D intake and stores are associated with lower rates of preterm births cesareans compared to women who are low in vitamin D! Vitamin D may help uterine function in labor.

The results of a randomized trial in South Carolina of a multiethnic pregnant population of more than six hundred women taking 4,000, 2,000, or 400 IU of vitamin D₃ were recently reported. The number of preterm births (at thirty-two and thirty-seven weeks' gestation) among women taking 4,000 IU were half that of those taking the currently recommended 400 IU dose, and the women had 30 percent less morbidities, including 25 percent fewer infections with no reported adverse effects.[4] A cross-sectional study by Merewood et al. that adjusted for demographic variables and alcohol use found that women who were vitamin D deficient (i.e., with less than 15 nanograms per milliliter [ng/ml]) were four times more likely to have a primary cesarean birth. The authors propose that adequate vitamin D is required for effective uterine function during labor.

Vitamin D aids in the absorption of calcium from the intestines and the breakdown and assimilation of phosphorous, both necessary for bone formation. It helps maintain a healthy nervous system, normal heart functioning, and normal clotting responses by helping the body absorb calcium. Deficiencies of this nutrient can lead to bone deformities, and excesses of it can lead to dizziness, nausea, and weakness, similar to what is experienced from overexposure to the sun.

Herbal sources include alfalfa and nettle.

### Vitamin E

This is another fat-soluble vitamin. The most common form is alpha-tocopherol, which literally means "the substance required to bring forth normal births." Vitamin E prevents the destruction of cells and vital nutrients, and it enables body tissue to function with less oxygen, thereby increasing endurance and stamina. It is essential to certain types of metabolism, aids in cell division, and promotes health and healing of body tissue. Vitamin E helps prevent abnormal blood clotting and is said to increase the pain threshold.

It is abundant in whole grains, nuts, oils, eggs, wheat germ, legumes, and green leafy vegetables. Vitamin E can be obtained from a diet rich in these foods, and from your prenatal vitamin. Additional supplementation is not recommended in pregnancy.

---

4. Hollis, BW, et al., "Vitamin D supplementation during pregnancy: double blind, randomized clinical trial of safety and effectiveness," *J Bone Miner Res* 26, no. 12 (Dec 2011): 2341-2357.

## MINERALS

### Calcium

The most abundant mineral in the body, calcium is needed in the formation of a baby's bones and teeth, and in maintaining the health of the mother's bones, teeth, and connective tissue. It is essential in controlling the coagulation of blood. Muscles cannot contract and release without it. Calcium helps maintain healthy nerves, normal metabolism, mineral balance throughout the body, and regular heartbeat. It is said to increase the pain threshold, and its effectiveness in promoting nerve and muscular relaxation prevents and reduces insomnia. Signs of calcium deficiency include irritability, insomnia, and leg cramps. Sources of calcium are milk, hard cheeses, yogurt, leafy green vegetables, almonds, sea vegetables, salmon, and blackstrap molasses. It is important to maintain a balance of calcium and phosphorus in the diet as excess of either will cause losses of both. Also, calcium and magnesium work together, and when you supplement calcium, take a supplement that contains both of these minerals. Be sure to eat four servings of calcium-rich foods each day.

Herbal sources include alfalfa, red clover, red raspberry leaves, nettle, chamomile, dandelion, kelp, and dulse.

### Magnesium

Magnesium is a highly abundant mineral in the earth—and in your body. It plays a role in all of your cells, helping them to make energy and regulating your metabolism, including your blood sugar. It also plays a key role in your nervous system, relaxes your muscles, and prevents spasms in your blood vessels. It also plays a role in the functioning of many of your important enzymes. Deficiency in pregnancy can be associated with preterm contractions and also preeclampsia. Many women find (contrary to lack of scientific evidence supporting this) that it is effective in treating restless leg syndrome. It is a safe option to try—usually 400 to 600 milligrams per day, taken before bed. Magnesium citrate can be used if you also have constipation; if not, use magnesium glycinate.

Some dietary sources rich in magnesium include pumpkin and sunflower seeds, millet, quinoa, almonds, spinach, Swiss chard, black beans, yogurt, peanut butter, oatmeal, and tofu.

### Iron

Many women enter pregnancy already low in iron. While iron deficiency anemia of the fetus is extremely rare, optimal iron availability adds to optimal oxygenation of fetal tissue. Adequate iron in pregnancy leads to building adequate iron stores for the newborn and also allows the mother to handle blood loss at birth more effectively, with less risk of postpartum anemia. Iron deficiency anemia can lead to fatigue, increased prenatal nausea, depression, shortness of breath, and restless leg syndrome in pregnancy, so getting ahead of the game by ensuring that the mother is not anemic *prior* to pregnancy can prevent some common pregnancy discomforts. Dietary sources of iron include these:

- Meats such as beef, pork, lamb, liver, and other organ meats

- Poultry such as chicken, duck, and turkey (especially dark meat)

- Sardines, anchovies, clams, mussels, and oysters (Check with your health care provider before consuming other types of fish as some may contain high levels of mercury.)

- Leafy greens including broccoli, kale, turnip greens, and collards

- Pinto, kidney, and black beans

- Dried apricots, black Mission figs, raisins, and prunes

- Blackstrap molasses

Care should be taken with the latter two options, as they are high in sugar. Red meats contain the most absorbable form of iron called *heme* iron. Vitamin C enhances iron absorption whereas calcium (including dairy products) interferes with it.

Herbal sources include nettle, dandelion, yellow dock, kelp, alfalfa, watercress, and fennel.

> *We tend to think that a baby in utero is entirely cut off from the world that lies just beyond a thin layer of skin. We seldom consider the child within as a conscious being, capable of responding to sounds and the inner environment the mother creates through her sense of well-being or lack of it.*
>
> —JOY GARDNER

### Iodine

Recent data shows that iodine levels in the United States have been decreasing. Iodine, which must be obtained from the diet or supplementation, is necessary for thyroid hormone production as well as fetal neurodevelopment. It is recommended that pregnant women supplement with 150 micrograms of potassium iodide daily. Iodine deficiency can lead to fertility problems; it is the primary cause of mental retardation in the world, and even mild deficiency in pregnant women can have an impact on the IQ of offspring. Thyroid problems are also very common in the postpartum period; adequate iodine supplementation may help prevent this problem. Iodine is widely undersupplemented in the United States, and thyroid problems are underdiagnosed.

Iodine is needed for the healthy function of the thyroid gland, which is responsible for the rate of metabolism, growth and development, and mental balance. Deficiency may be signaled by frequent infections, weakness, nervous system problems, and low activity levels.

Iodine is found in seafood—fish and sea vegetables (kelp or kombu, dulse, alaria or wakame, hijiki, and nori)—and in iodized salt and sea salt. A few vegetables contain small amounts of iodine.

Herbal sources include watercress, kelp, dulse, and Irish moss.

### Phosphorus

Usually found in abundance in most diets, phosphorus is important for bone development, healthy teeth, and the healthy growth of fetal cells.

Herbal sources include alfalfa, red raspberry leaves, dandelion, watercress, caraway seeds, and comfrey. Legumes, pumpkin seeds, and salmon are food sources rich in phosphorous. It is generally not hard to obtain in a well-balanced diet.

### Zinc

Zinc is essential for normal immune system functioning, healthy hormone production, organ development, healthy reproduction, and release of vitamin A from the liver. It also protects the bones and joints as well as the prostate gland and sexual fluids in males.

Food sources include oysters, other shellfish, herring, nuts, seeds, beef, eggs, chicken, turkey, fruits, and vegetables.

Herbal sources include watercress.

### Sodium

Sodium is an essential mineral for maintaining health during pregnancy. It is necessary for maintaining both fluid and electrolyte balance as well as preventing muscular irritability. It is available in common salt, sea salt, and many foods. Pregnant women should reduce their consumption of junk foods, which are heavily salted, but should salt their other foods to taste using a natural form of salt such as sea salt.

*Growing a baby is a big job that requires you to have good materials, enough to meet your needs and your baby's.* 

### Other Minerals

Other minerals, such as potassium, which is needed for strong muscle contraction, and many trace minerals should all be available to you in your diet if you are eating the quantity and variety of foods already mentioned.

## ESSENTIAL FATTY ACIDS

Essential fatty acids (EFAs) are critical and overlooked nutrients needed for optimal brain development in the fetus. The breast milk of mothers in the United States is among the lowest in essential fatty acids in the world, indicating that pregnant women in this country are likely very deficient in EFAs, as are their babies. Inadequate intake of EFAs has been associated with decreased mental development, increased rates of allergies and asthma, and other atopic diseases. Essential fatty acids are found in high amounts in walnuts and walnut oil; flaxseeds and flaxseed oil; deepwater fish such as salmon, tuna, and cod; and avocados. During pregnancy, if one chooses to supplement, it is advisable to use both an evening primrose oil supplement and a high-quality fish oil supplement in order to get a balance of both omega-3 and omega-6 fatty acids. It is not necessary to supplement with fish oil if fish is eaten as a regular part of the weekly diet. However, the American Academy of Pediatrics and the American Academy of Obstetrics and Gynecology do recommend that pregnant women not consume deep sea fish more than once or twice weekly to avoid excessive consumption of mercury contamination from fish, which may be transferred to the developing fetus.

# Vegetarian and Other Natural Foods Diets

There are four common variations on the basic vegetarian diet: the vegetarian who occasionally eats fish or chicken, but relies primarily on nonmeat sources for nutrients; the lacto-ovo vegetarian who eats no meats but does eat dairy products and eggs; the lacto vegetarian who eats dairy but no meats or eggs; and the vegan who includes absolutely no animal products in the diet whatsoever and frequently excludes honey as well.

A person on a macrobiotic diet eats whole grains, beans, vegetables, occasional fruits in season, sea vegetables, seeds, and nuts, with the occasional inclusion of fish. Such a person relies on the concept of yin and yang to create balanced menus to meet individual health needs and create harmony in the body, mind, and spirit.

A person on a raw-food diet believes that humans, like animals, should eat foods in a raw state. Emphasis is placed on fruits, vegetables, fresh juices, sprouts, nuts, and seeds (preferably sprouted). The idea is that cooked foods cause impurities in the body.

It is possible to meet your nutritional needs on any of these diets during pregnancy if you give close attention to meeting these needs. Vegetarian diets that include a variety of foods are likely to include much less fat as well as fewer, if any, chemical additives and fewer overprocessed foods. Be open to your needs and don't get stuck on a preconceived idea. Respect your intuition whether you are a vegetarian wanting a piece of chicken, a vegan wanting a cheese sandwich, or a macrobiotic wanting a grapefruit in the middle of winter in Boston. The danger lies in becoming an extremist and in excluding foods that might be just what your body needs. Of course there are many vegetarian ways to meet your needs if you choose to be strictly vegetarian—you must be willing to educate yourself about your nutritional needs—and always listen to your body over dogma!

Many natural foods diets are based on the idea that the body is dirty and needs cleansing through fasting. This is untrue and potentially very dangerous for pregnant women. Our bodies are capable of digesting meat, dairy products (unless a specific intolerance exists), and other foods often considered taboo. The key is moderation and balance. Also, foods serve different purposes. For example, fruits and raw foods cool us down and promote elimination while heavy carbohydrates and proteins warm us and help us to build our bodies. We must recognize what is appropriate for different seasons of the year and of our lives. Pregnancy is a time of building and nourishing, with elimination being an essential function for health, but not our primary goal.

Women who eat a healthy, well-balanced vegetarian diet may in fact enjoy a healthier pregnancy than women who rely heavily on the standard American diet, which is laden with sugar and fat and excludes fresh vegetables, whole grains, legumes, nuts, and seeds. The primary concern for vegetarian women is that they get ample protein; also, if dairy is not eaten, foods containing calcium should be plentiful in the diet. There are many foods that can provide these nutrients, and, in fact, in China where almost no dairy is used and a lot of dark green vegetables are consumed, the women have the lowest osteoporosis rates in the world. See "Calcium" earlier in this chapter, and refer to the Bibliography for more information on calcium substitutes. I encourage women not to drink milk during pregnancy and to rely instead on nondairy calcium sources, as well as hard cheeses and active-culture yogurt.

To obtain adequate protein from a vegetarian diet, these women must learn to combine their protein sources to create complete proteins, as discussed earlier in this section. There are various ways this can be done:

- Grains (rice, corn, wheat, millet, oats, rye, barley, and so on) can be combined with a slightly smaller amount of beans or legumes (lentils, peanuts, garbanzo beans, kidney beans, pinto beans, black beans, azuki beans, navy beans, soybeans, and so on).

- Grains can be combined with dairy products.

- Nuts and seeds can be combined with beans or legumes.

A few examples of complete proteins include rice and beans; macaroni and cheese; rice and tahini (sesame seed paste); pasta with peanut sauce; granola that contains oats, peanuts, and sunflower seeds; whole-wheat bread with peanut butter; and tofu on toast. You don't need to eat complete proteins every time you have a protein food, but you should get four to five servings of complete proteins each day. I have enjoyed three completely vegetarian pregnancies, and one mostly vegetarian one. In my last pregnancy, I was inclined to eat fish and chicken, and so I occasionally added these foods (organic poultry only) to my diet. The main advantage for me in including dairy as a regular part of my diet was the fact that it is easy to prepare and is a filling source of energy. One can eat rice, beans, and cheese, for example, and feel more filled than by eating rice and beans alone. Yogurt, or cheese and crackers, makes a great, filling, quick snack. Also, dairy foods are complete proteins, so I didn't have to be as concerned about combining foods as I would on a vegan diet. It takes a larger quantity of vegetarian foods to satisfy the appetite than, say, a small piece of steak, but vegetarian food is also easier to digest and not likely to result in problems such as constipation or weight gain due to the high-fiber, low-fat nature of the foods.

I recommend that pregnant women do not drink milk because babies of mothers who drink a lot of milk tend to grow very big. I feel that this is a disadvantage in birthing. Milk molecules are also hard to digest, milk is high in fat, and it also contains hormones, both naturally occurring in cows and sometimes added with cattle feed. These hormones are not beneficial to human health and may possibly be harmful.

If you are pregnant and vegetarian, I can't overemphasize how important it is to eat a wide variety of foods in order to obtain all of the nutrients you now require. I've met many well-educated vegetarians whose diets were limited to just a few foods. Some rely on packaged foods. Processing is processing—it robs foods of nutrients. Also, many vegetarian women eat a lot of fruit and drink a lot of fruit juices, filling up on empty calories. Just being a vegetarian does not ensure that you are eating a healthy diet—it may mean merely that you are not eating unhealthy foods! If you plan to raise your child as a vegetarian, now is the time to do the research and feed yourself and your baby well.

# Cravings

As long as you are meeting all of your daily needs with healthy food, there is no reason that you should not enjoy an *occasional* pleasure food. Problems may arise when your craving is a result of poor nutrition or sugar or carbohydrate addiction, and you indulge the craving rather than going for the healthy food. For example, if you work outside the home while you are pregnant and find yourself craving a chocolate bar at 11:00 a.m. each day, your body is really telling you that you need energy. Instead of the calorie-dense but nutrient-empty candy bar, you could carry a healthy snack with you to work, such as a container of yogurt and some granola, apples and almond butter, hummus and vegetable sticks, nuts, or a nutritious high-protein low-sugar energy bar such as a KIND bar, and eat this when you feel the craving.

Frequently, cravings are specific clues about our nutritional needs. Deciphering them may take a bit of detective work. Frequently, a craving for sweets is a physical need for more protein in the diet. Try to replace junk foods with wholesome choices, and see how this affects your cravings. If you're eating well and still want some ice cream, bon appétit!

# Weight Gain—How Much?

We live in culture that equates thinness with success, beauty, and health. As a result, one in five women has an eating disorder, and many who have an eating disorder are of childbearing age. Many women are so out of touch with their bodies that they don't even know when they are hungry, a result of suppressing their instinctual, life-preserving urge to eat. What often happens is that women try to get by on as little food as possible, living in a state of hypoglycemia, frequently overloading on sugar and carbohydrates to restore their low blood sugar level to a semblance of normality. Thus, eating during pregnancy—and the need to gain weight—can be really tough for a lot of women.

Conversely, the growing prevalence of overweight and obese women of childbearing age is a major public health problem in the United States. Women who are overweight (BMI 25–30) and obese (BMI ≥30) are at greater risk of adverse reproductive health outcomes compared to women of optimal weight status. And because women are also more likely to retain gestational weight with each pregnancy, the problem compounds with each additional pregnancy. Obesity is entirely preventable. Gestational diabetes is as well. Sadly, a rapidly increasing number of women are entering pregnancy *already* obese.

And what is the medical response to pregnant women who are overweight? Restrict prenatal weight gain! No attention is paid to the *types* and *quality* of foods eaten, nor to actual nutrition, just to calorie restriction to limit weight gain. Yet food is information! So simply restricting weight gain does not mean that a woman is getting optimal—or even adequate—nutrition.

How much weight you gain in pregnancy is determined by your height and how much you weigh when you get pregnant. These two measures go into what it called your Body Mass Index (BMI). To calculate this, you can go to www.nhlbi.nih.gov /guidelines/obesity/BMI/bmicalc.htm but here is an overview:

- If you are underweight (with BMI less than 18.5),
  gain 8 to 40 pounds (12.5 to 18 kilograms)

- If you are a normal weight (with BMI equal to 18.5 to 24.9),
  gain 25 to 35 pounds (11.5 to 16 kilograms)

- If you are overweight (with BMI equal to 25.0 to 29.9),
  gain 15 to 25 pounds (7 to 11.5 kilograms)

- If you are obese (with BMI equal to greater than 30.0),
  gain 11 to 20 pounds (5 to 9 kilograms)

Weight gain within these parameters is associated with a lower rate of cesarean delivery, fewer infants with growth restriction or macrosomia, and a decreased incidence of postpartum obesity. Only 30 to 40 percent of pregnant women achieve appropriate weight gain. Undernutrition is also a huge risk: dieting during pregnancy is never recommended, even for morbidly obese women.

The amount you gain per week also varies by starting BMI, and there are some recommended variations based on race (for example, Asian women have different needs than white women or Latina or African American women). Weight gain also varies by trimester.

In the first trimester, you really don't need to gain much of anything to meet your baby's needs, so put your worries aside if you've been feeling sick, nauseated, and unable to eat much (or much of anything) healthy!

In the second and third trimesters, your appetite is probably better. You can expect to gain about 1 pound per week for women who are underweight or normal weight, 0.6 pounds for women who are overweight, and 0.5 pounds for women who are obese.

More important than stepping on the scale, however, is eating well and choosing from the right selection of foods. A steadily and properly growing baby is the most important thing. The scale doesn't tell us whether the baby is being nourished properly on healthy food. We do know that all kinds of food habits start in mom's womb, ranging from food preferences to quality of fat cells that can set the trend for healthy weight versus obesity!

The bottom line is to listen to your body, pay attention to your hunger signals, and learn to choose healthy foods.

Let your intuition guide you in your food choices. If your intuition tells you to eat a piece of salmon though you are an ardent vegetarian, you may choose your intuited needs over your ideals. Similarly, if you dislike collard greens but your body says "greens," you may have to develop a taste for collards and find a few delicious recipes! To develop this intuition, allow yourself to be very still and quiet and suspend your conscious mind for a few minutes to allow messages to arise from your right brain or intuitive mode of thinking. And then simply ask yourself or the baby what you need. Make a note of what you imagine the answer to be. Try this each day for a week and follow through on the messages that you receive. Eat for nutrition and pleasure, and you will meet your needs. Enjoyment of food is one of the most important keys to good digestion, which must also occur if you are going to absorb and utilize the foods you do eat.

## Take Inventory

A great way to see if your current way of eating is giving you the nutrition you need is to create a three-day food journal. Write down everything you eat and drink for three days, including anything not healthy, to get a true picture of your nutrition. Then bring the food journal to your midwife or a trusted nutritionist for review. Just the act of writing down your food intake for yourself can be really enlightening and informative—you will likely realize how you can improve the quality of your nutrition. Then reviewing it with someone else can give you the guidance you need to add and take away those items that are—or aren't—optimally healthy. Another set of knowledgeable eyes can also help you identify why you might be having various food cravings, sugar crashes, fatigue, constipation, anemia, or other symptoms you might be chalking up to "normal pregnancy complaints" that are actually based on your nutrition! Hello, more fiber; good-bye, constipation!

# Foods to Avoid in Pregnancy

Fish is a wonderful protein and omega-3 fatty acid–containing food source, but, as mentioned, you should keep mercury and chemical content in mind. Large fish that are high on the food chain and have long lives are also more likely to have accumulated a lot of mercury; too much mercury can harm baby's brain and nerves, especially during development. Some fish may also contain cancer-causing chemicals such as dioxins and polychlorinated biphenyls (PCBs). In general, avoid farm-raised fish and eat only low-mercury fish during pregnancy including blue crab (mid-Atlantic), flounder, salmon (wild Pacific), sardines, and shrimp. Completely avoid shark, swordfish, king mackerel, tilefish, tuna steaks, canned tuna, sea bass, Gulf Coast oysters, marlin, halibut, pike, walleye, white croaker, and largemouth bass.

## WHAT ABOUT SUSHI?

Raw fish should not be eaten as it may contain parasites (germs) that could harm you or your baby. Vegetarian sushi is totally fine, but if it is prepared along with raw fish, contamination with parasites remains a risk.

## WHAT ABOUT RAW MILK AND CHEESE?

As you go organic, you may hear that unpasteurized dairy is closer to natural. While this may be true, unpasteurized dairy can contain a bacteria that can cause a disease called *listeriosis*, which may cause miscarriage, stillbirth, or serious health problems for your baby. During pregnancy, you should avoid soft cheeses like Mexican-style queso blanco, queso fresco, feta, Camembert, blue cheeses, or Brie if it is made with unpasteurized milk. Read the label and do not eat the cheese if the label says it is made with raw milk or unpasteurized milk. If it is made with pasteurized milk and kept in the refrigerator at 40°F or less, it is safe to eat. Similarly, it is best to drink pasteurized juices during pregnancy unless you are making them fresh at home yourself.

> **CAUTION: Read the label and do not eat the cheese if the label says it is made with raw milk or unpasteurized milk.**

Also, make sure your meats are well cooked, and be careful with alfalfa sprouts because they have been known to cause salmonella infection.

# CHAPTER 6

# Herbs, Safety, and Pregnancy Health

*The desire to avoid unnecessary interventions* as well as an inclination toward what is natural has led many pregnant women to seek alternatives, for example, the use of herbs, for the treatment of common pregnancy complaints. Studies and surveys estimate that up to 45 percent of women have used herbs during pregnancy.

## Are Herbs Safe During Pregnancy?

Herbs have been used for the treatment of discomforts and problems arising during pregnancy and childbirth dating at least back to ancient Egypt. Childbearing women commonly experience minor complaints for which the use of natural remedies may be gentler and safer than over-the-counter and prescription pharmaceuticals. Little is known scientifically about the risk of using herbs during pregnancy, as most have not been formally evaluated and ethical considerations limit human clinical investigation during pregnancy. Much the same can be said for the use of many pharmaceuticals during pregnancy.

Most of what is currently known about botanical use during pregnancy is based on a significant body of historical, empirical, and observational evidence, and limited pharmacologic and animal studies. Overall, most herbs have a high safety profile with little evidence of harm. Few adverse events have been reported, and those that have been have typically involved the consumption of known toxic herbs, adulterations, or inappropriate use or dosage of botanical therapies. However, lack of proof of harm is not synonymous with proof of safety. Some of the harmful effects of herbs may not be readily apparent until after use has been discontinued or may only occur with cumulative use. While gentle herbs and simple home remedies have a long historical track record of safety, pregnant women are increasingly seeking advice from sources that may not always be reliable (for example, via the Internet), and they may also be trying to treat potentially serious problems than can arise during the childbearing cycle.

Schools of thought differ on whether herbs should be used routinely during pregnancy. Some believe that because most are not proven safe during pregnancy, they should be entirely avoided, while others see certain herbs more as foods that can provide additional sources of nutrition during pregnancy, or as tonics that can encourage and support optimal pregnancy health and uterine function. Perhaps the most reasonable approach to herb safety is a risk-benefit approach that compares the safety of the individual herb and the severity of the symptom/condition to the safety of the corresponding conventional medical approach. Certain signs and symptoms arising during pregnancy *always* warrant medical attention and should *not* be treated with herbs. See "Warning and Danger Signs uring Pregnancy," page 79.

# Using Herbs During Pregnancy

The most prudent approach to the use of herbs during pregnancy is to avoid herbs during the first trimester unless medically indicated (i.e., nausea and vomiting of pregnancy [NVP], threatened miscarriage), and after the first trimester, to use herbs that are known either scientifically or historically to be safe during pregnancy. Beverages and nutritive teas that are known to be safe in moderate amounts (i.e., red raspberry, spearmint, chamomile, lemon balm, nettles, rose hips) and ingestion of normal amounts of cooking spices are considered generally safe enough to be used freely.

There are many herbs that contain mostly benign, nutritive substances such as carbohydrates, vitamins, and minerals. Herbs such as nettles (*Urtica dioica*), milky oats (*Avena sativa*), and red raspberry leaf (*Rubus idaeus*) are examples. Several herbs have also been demonstrated scientifically to be safe during pregnancy (see the table "Herbs Considered Safe in Pregnancy," page 80).

On the other hand, there are numerous herbs that for safety reasons should not be used at all. Extensive lists of these are available.[1, 2] Also see the table "Herb

---

1. Aviva Romm, *Botanical Medicine for Women's Health* (St. Louis, Mo.: Churchill Livingstone/Elsevier, 2010).

2. Zoë Gardner and Michael McGuffin, *American Herbal Products Association's Botanical Safety Handbook* (Boca Raton, FL: CRC Press, 2013).

Contraindicated for Use in Pregnancy" (page 89); it condenses this information, presenting the most important therapeutic categories and representative herbs to avoid.

Somewhere between the categories of herbs considered to be safe and those that should not be used at all are those herbs that are not appropriate to use for daily or routine intake, but that can be used, if necessary, for brief or more extended periods of time for specific conditions. For example, licorice, if used short term for a sore throat, say—and for no longer than a week—may be entirely safe and appropriate; however, it is contraindicated for patients with hypertension. Further, long-term use of even licorice candy containing actual licorice extract has been associated with preterm birth.

During pregnancy, you should consult an herbalist, midwife, or physician trained in the use of botanicals when using herbs medically (i.e., to treat a specific symptom or condition) rather than simply nutritively or as a general pregnancy tonic (as one would use red raspberry leaf or nettles).

In addition to common complaints of pregnancy, pregnant and lactating women are subject to the run-of-the-mill complaints and illnesses we all face—colds, indigestion, headache, and so on, for which they may seek herbal care. Many of these problems can be addressed safely and gently with mild herbs such as echinacea, ginger, or chamomile, respectively.

Many herbs are both safe and highly effective as remedies for common health complaints, and herbs and spices are consumed daily around the world by pregnant women as a natural part of the diet. Taken in small amounts and using only herbs that are known to be safe during pregnancy, they can provide relief for many minor pregnancy complaints. In expert hands, many herbs can also be used for more serious conditions, including complex pregnancy-related problems.

**Caution: While many herbal remedies are gentle and safe, herbs are also pharmacologically active and potent medicinal agents, and therefore great care and caution is advised for their use during pregnancy.**

**Whenever possible, the use of herbs should be avoided during the first trimester; if it is necessary to use herbs during this time, only those herbs with no known teratogenic, mutagenic, or abortifacient properties should be used, and only in the lowest possible doses.**

It is important to remember that while the human species has a long history of using herbs safely, very few studies have been done to demonstrate the safety and effectiveness of herbs during pregnancy. Consider the following key points:

- *Natural* is not synonymous with *harmless* or *safe*—many botanical medicines contain potent pharmacological substances.

- Many herbal constituents are capable of passing through the placenta and can therefore directly affect the fetus.

- Physiological and metabolic changes during pregnancy may influence the action of herbs in the body.

- Unless medically indicated, avoid use of herbs (and drugs) during the first trimester.

- Preventive treatment and early intervention with herbs is safer and more effective than treating advanced problems, since dosage can typically be minimized and gentler herbs applied early on.

- Know each herb you are considering using by clearly understanding side effects and contraindications for pregnant women.

**Warning and Danger Signs During Pregnancy: Seek Medical Attention!**
- Persistent vaginal bleeding
- *Initial* outbreak of herpes blisters during the first trimester
- Severe pelvic or abdominal pain
- Persistent, severe midback pain
- Edema of the hands and face
- Severe headaches, blurry vision, or epigastric (the area under the center of your ribcage) pain
- Rupture of membranes prior to thirty-seven weeks of pregnancy
- Regular uterine contractions prior to thirty-seven weeks of pregnancy
- Cessation of fetal movement

# Herbs Considered Safe in Pregnancy [3, 4, 5, 6, 7, 8]

The following table provides an overview of a number of herbs that have been demonstrated to be safe for use during pregnancy through clinical trials or scientific evaluation of safety.

> WARNING: If you are unsure about the safety of an herb during pregnancy, do not use it.

| BOTANICAL NAME | REASON FOR USE | CLINICAL TRIALS IN PREGNANCY | TYPICAL DAILY DOSE | COMMENTS |
|---|---|---|---|---|
| Red raspberry leaf<br><br>*Rubus idaeus* | Mineral-rich nutritive tonic<br><br>Uterine tonic that promotes an expedient labor with minimal bleeding<br><br>Also an astringent for diarrhea | Positive | 1.5 to 5 grams per day in tea or infusion | Highly astringent herbs can, theoretically, interfere with intestinal nutrient absorption. |
| Echinacea<br><br>*Echinacea* spp. | Reduces duration and recurrence of colds and upper respiratory tract infections (URI) | Positive | 5 to 20 milliliters tincture | The dose listed here and considered safe by herbalists is higher than that used in the study by Gallo et al. |
| Ginger<br><br>*Zingiber officinalis* | Antinauseant, antiemetic<br><br>Used for NVP, *hyperemesis gravidarum, and general nausea* | Positive | Up to 1 gram dried powder per day | Higher doses of ginger are traditionally considered emmenagogic, meaning they bring on the menses.<br><br>Untreated *hyperemesis gravidarum* in pregnancy can cause serious adverse outcomes. |
| Cranberry<br><br>*Vaccinium macrocarpon* | Prevents and relieves urinary tract infection (UTI) | None identified | 16 to 32 fluid ounces of juice per day | Untreated UTI in pregnancy can cause serious adverse outcomes. |
| Chamomile<br><br>*Matricaria Recutita* | Promotes general relaxation<br><br>Treats insomnia<br><br>Treats flatulence | None identified | 1 to 5 grams per day in tea | No scientifically proven contraindications. |

Because the practice of herbal medicine is unregulated in the United States, anyone, whether or not they have training in herbs, can give advice on their use. This includes doctors, nurses, and midwives who may have the best of intentions but not the best information. A qualified herbalist or a health professional specially trained in the use of herbs during pregnancy (a midwife, nurse, or physician who has done specific research in this area; a licensed naturopathic physician who has graduated from a four-year naturopathic college; or a registered Chinese herbalist) can provide you with safety information. You can also contact several of the organizations that exist to provide consumers with herbal safety information, for example, the American Botanical Council.

It is not hard to learn how to incorporate herbs into your daily life, but it is essential that you choose from those that are known to be safe during pregnancy. The best way to benefit from herbs is to use them regularly as a source of nourishment— not only when you are ill or uncomfortable. There are many herbs that can be used safely during pregnancy that not only provide additional vitamins and minerals to your diet, but also strengthen the womb, liver, nervous system, digestive system, and urogenital tract. Herbs derive nutrients from the soil that many of our common foods may lack. Herbs are relatively inexpensive, particularly if you buy them in bulk. Tea drinking is one way to incorporate herbs into your routine. It is a daily custom in many parts of the world and can provide a nourishing ritual during your pregnancy.

The herbs mentioned in this book can be considered safe in pregnancy as indicated by generations of safe usage, as well as by clinical studies when available. Known exceptions are noted. However, there are a few potential problems that should always be kept in mind:

- **No two people are exactly alike, and therefore you cannot know in advance the exact effect an herb will have on your body (or your baby).** It is best to rely on tried-and-true herbs during pregnancy and to begin with small amounts, gradually increasing dosage as appropriate and necessary. For example, chamomile is an herb considered completely

3. M. Simpson et al., "Raspberry Leaf in Pregnancy: Its Safety and Efficacy in Labor," *Journal of Midwifery & Women's Health* 46, no. 2 (March–April 2001): 51–59.

4. Myra Parsons et al., "Raspberry Leaf and Its Effect on Labour: Safety and Efficacy," *Australian College of Midwives Journal* 12, no. 3 (September 1999): 20–25.

5. M. Gallo et al., "Pregnancy Outcome Following Exposure to Echinacea: A Prospective Controlled Study," *Archives of Internal Medicine* 160, no. 20 (November 2000): 3141–3143.

6. W. Fischer-Rasmussen et al., "Ginger Treatment of Hyperemesis Gravidarum," *European Journal of Obstetrics, Gynecology, and Reproductive Biology* 38, no. 1 (4 January 1991): 19–24.

7. T. Vutyavanich et al., "Ginger for Nausea and Vomiting in Pregnancy: Randomized, Doublemasked, Placebo-controlled Trial," *Obstetrics and Gynecology* 97, no. 4 (April 2001): 577–582.

8. T. Low Dog, *Women's Health in Complementary and Integrative Medicine: A Clinical Guide* (St. Louis, MO: Elsevier, 2004).

safe and free from any toxic side effects according to extensive German research, yet because of its membership in the *Compositae* family, along with herbs such as ragweed, a rare individual may have an allergic reaction to it. With all herbs, it is wise to proceed slowly and carefully.

- **There is always a risk of contamination, adulteration, or substitution of one plant species for another in commerce.** For example, in one instance, a Canadian mother thought she was taking an herb, *Eleutherococcus senticosus*, considered fairly safe for use during pregnancy. After taking the capsule product regularly during the pregnancy, she gave birth to a baby with congenital androgenism—the baby was hirsute (covered with an unnatural amount of hair). Upon scientific analysis of the product that the woman was taking, it was determined that it contained *Periploca*, another herb entirely. *Periploca* is not considered safe for use during pregnancy. It is very important to purchase herbs from reliable sources only. If you are unsure, contact an experienced herbalist in your community, or one of the national botanical medicine associations, such as the American Herbalists Guild (see Resources).

- **If you are harvesting plants yourself from the wild, make sure that you are identifying them correctly. Confusing the desired herb with a poisonous plant can be a fatal mistake—and one that is not that hard to make.** Even if you purchase fresh herbs from someone who has harvested them, make sure they know their stuff. I recently heard the story of an experienced harvester who came upon a group of people harvesting herbs in the woods for inclusion in commercial products. They thought they were harvesting a medicinal herb commonly used in many products but were inadvertently harvesting poisonous water hemlock. Fortunately, the more experienced passerby herbalist informed them of their mistake before it was too late.

- **When purchasing bulk herbs, be certain that the common names and the Latin names of the plants correlate with each other so you know that you are getting what you are looking for** (see appendix B). Plants have many different common names, but their Latin names are internationally accepted as a standard.

- **Be certain to take herbal tinctures, pills, and capsules from carefully labeled jars so that no mistakes are made.** Again, this is especially important during pregnancy and with young children.

- **It is essential to follow general dosage guidelines for each herb.** The idea that more is better is dangerous when applied to any medication, including herbs. Although most herbs are very gentle, their effects should not be underestimated. In appendix A, Herbal Preparations, you will find general dosage guidelines. Specific guidelines accompany all herbal protocols discussed in the context of conditions later in this book.

- **Herbs that you take during pregnancy will usually affect your baby as well as you.** Herbs contain potent chemical substances, many of which have demonstrable effects on the body. Certain herbs, for example, contain volatile oils or alkaloids that can affect the functioning of the central nervous system and, when taken during the first trimester of pregnancy, can interfere with the development of the baby's nervous system. Other herbs have what are known as *emmenagogic* properties— that is, they stimulate pelvic circulation. While this may be desirable when a woman is close to the time of birth, the result earlier in the pregnancy might be the stimulation of contractions, perhaps even premature labor.

- **Pregnancy is a natural process, and, unless you are ill, it is unnecessary to use herbs other than as gentle toners and nourishment.**

- **If you are ill and wish to use herbs remedially, it is essential that you avoid herbs that are contraindicated during pregnancy, particularly during the first trimester.** Use herbs only according to recommended times and dosages.

- **Consult an experienced herbalist when you are unsure about the safety of using a particular herb during pregnancy.**

> *A woman is the full circle, within her is the power—to create, nurture, and transform.*
>
> —DIANE MARIECHILD

## Herbs to Avoid During Pregnancy

The table that accompanies this section lists those herbs most commonly contraindicated for internal use during pregnancy. For a more exhaustive list, see the *Botanical Safety Handbook* by McGuffin et al. (1997). [9]

There are some herbs on the list below that may be used in small quantities for certain conditions, where the risks of using the herb are outweighed by the

---

9. Gardner and McGuffin, *Botanical Safety Handbook.*

benefits, *but only with qualified supervision*. An example of this would be the use of very small amounts of goldenseal for severe diarrhea during midpregnancy, if diarrhea was causing the mother to lose weight and become dehydrated. However, large doses of goldenseal during early pregnancy may be unsafe for the developing embryo.

Also, certain herbs that are contraindicated by Western herbalists and Western scientific research for use during pregnancy are regularly used in other countries, such as *dong quai*, which is prescribed as a blood tonic for pregnant women in

## Herbs Contraindicated for Use in Pregnancy

Alder buckthorn, *Rhamnus frangula*

Aloe, *Aloe vera*

Angelica, *Angelica archangelica*

Arnica, *Arnica montana*

Autumn crocus, *Colchicum autumnale*

Barberry, *Berberis vulgaris*

Beth root, *Trillium spp.*

Blessed thistle, *Cnicus benedictus*

Blood root, *Sanguinaria canadensis*

Blue cohosh, *Caulophyllum thalictroides*

Broom, *Sarpthamnus scoparius*

Butternut, *Juglans canadensis*

Calamus, *Acorus calamus*

Calendula, *Calendula officinalis*

Cascara sagrada, *Rhamnus purshiana*

Coltsfoot, *Tussilago farfara*

Comfrey, *Symphytum officinale*

Cotton root, *Gossypium herbaceum*

Cowslip, *Primula veris*

Damiana, *Turnera aphrodisiaca*

Ephedra (*ma huang*), *Ephedra vulgaris*

Feverfew, *Tanacetum parthenium*

Ginseng, *Panax quinquefolium*

Goat's rue, *Galega officinalis*

Goldenseal, *Hydrastis canadensis*

Gotu kola, *Hydrocotyle asiatica*

Ipecac, *Ipecac ipechachuana*

Juniper berries, *Juniperis communis*

Licorice, *Glycyrrhiza glabra*

Lily of the valley, *Convallaria magalis*

Lobelia, *Lobelia inflata*

Male fern, *Dryopteris filix-mas*

Mandrake, *Podophyllum peltatum*

Mistletoe, *Viscum album*

Mugwort, *Artemesia vulgare*

Nutmeg, *Myristica officinalis*
(small amounts fine)

Osha, *Ligusticum porten*

Parsley, *Petroselinum crispum*
(small amounts fine)

Pennyroyal, *Mentha pulegium*

Periwinkle, *Vinca spp.*

Peruvian bark, *Cinchona spp.*

Pleurisy root, *Aesclepius tuberosa*

Poke root, *Phytolacca decondra*

Rhubarb, *Rheum palmatum*

Rue, *Ruta graveolens*

Sage, *Salvia officinalis*

Sarsaparilla, *Smilax officinalis*

Shepherd's purse, *Capsella bursa-pastoris*

Stillingia, *Stillingia sylvatica*

Tansy, *Tanacetum vulgare*

Thuja, *Thuja occidentalis*

Wormwood, *Artemesia absinthum*

Yarrow, *Achillea millefolium*

China. It is wise to use such herbs cautiously, if at all, during pregnancy if you do not have prior herbal knowledge or the assistance of an herbalist. *Pregnancy is not a good time to experiment with generally contraindicated herbs.* Further, Chinese herbs, especially prepared products known as "patent products," are notoriously contaminated with herbs not listed on the package—sometimes with pharmaceutical medications and even heavy metals. These should be avoided during pregnancy unless prescribed by a qualified herbalist or Chinese doctor familiar with clean, safe brands.

Specific categories of herbs are known to be contraindicated during pregnancy:

- One group of herbs that has come under scrutiny are those containing pyrrolizidine alkaloids (PAs). These are known to cause liver damage in both adults and developing fetuses. Comfrey, coltsfoot, and borage are the main culprits, containing varying amounts of these PAs. It is therefore most prudent to avoid the internal use of these herbs other than very occasionally and only after the first trimester of pregnancy.

    CAUTION: **External use of comfrey in small amounts for a short duration is probably safe, but PAs can cross the skin, so they should not be used for prolonged periods on broken skin.**

- Herbs that contain other strong alkaloids (often recognizable by their strongly bitter taste), whether they be those that strongly promote digestive functions and metabolism or those that perform other duties such as enhancing cardiac function, are to be avoided during pregnancy. Choices of gentle herbs can be applied for improving digestion.

- Laxative herbs that exert their effects by strongly promoting bowel peristalsis can also promote uterine contractions and so should be avoided during pregnancy. Gentler methods of promoting bowel functioning should be used, such as dietary changes, exercise, and bulk laxatives (e.g., flaxseed).

- Herbs with strong hormonal activity and those known to promote menstruation (known as *emmenagogues*) are to be avoided completely. Strong herbs used specifically to destroy intestinal worms are contraindicated as is the internal use of all essential oils.

- Certain herbs may be considered for use during labor, but only with the guidance of an experienced midwife or physician.

# What Forms of Herbs Are Safe During Pregnancy?

The forms in which herbs are administered (i.e., tincture, tea) can affect their strength and efficacy. Use water-based extracts (teas, infusion) to minimize extraction of bioactive compounds or to avoid excessive consumption of alcohol in an alcohol-based preparations, which are also typically more medicinally concentrated products. External applications, including vaginal use (i.e., for the treatment of vaginal infections) of most herbs are considered safe; however, some herbs (for example, poke root, pennyroyal oil, and thuja) that are known to be toxic should be avoided internally and topically.

Herbs can provide substantial relief for common complaints and concerns that arise during pregnancy and childbirth. The power of herbs should be respected during pregnancy, and therefore, they should be used with caution. However, many herbs may be contraindicated on the basis of very limited findings, erroneous reports, or by association with a problem rather than a proven causal effect. Many herbs that have not been evaluated may, nonetheless, offer simple, safe, gentle, and effective solutions for many common pregnancy problems ranging from anemia to vaginitis. Good diet and nutrition, exercise, and healthful lifestyle including a positive outlook and strong social support are the cornerstones of an optimal childbearing experience.

## Nourishment Tea 🌿

This is my favorite beverage in pregnancy. It is a nutrient supplement (iron, calcium, and many vitamins and trace minerals) and birth preparation brew. The dried herbs can be mixed in a large batch to have on hand. The tea is delicious both hot and cold, and it can be enjoyed by your whole family. You can vary the quantities of the ingredients or add and omit herbs from time to time. It is safe to drink this brew throughout the second and third trimester of pregnancy and during labor. It is beneficial for the postpartum as well, as it helps with milk production.

- 2 parts red raspberry leaf
- 2 parts nettle
- 1/2 part rose hips
- 1/4 part spearmint leaf

Mix all of the dried herbs together and store in an airtight container away from heat and light. To prepare your infusion, place a heaping 1/4 cup of the mixture in a quart-size jar. Add boiling water to fill the jar, cover, and let steep for a minimum of thirty minutes and a maximum of two hours. Strain, sweeten, and drink one to four cups daily.

# CHAPTER 7

# Exercise and Posture

➤➤➤❬❬❬

*Exercise is vitally important* for health in pregnancy. It increases circulation, which promotes well-being and prevents depression; it helps oxygenate the blood, reducing fatigue; it prevents the buildup of tension in the muscles; it reduces pelvic congestion and thus cramping, low backache, ligament pain, and constipation; and it prevents congestion of blood in the lower extremities, reducing leg cramps and tension as well as varicosities. Exercise promotes tone in the muscles, making the body ready for birth, aids recovery of organ tone and placement after birth, and also prevents prolapse of the pelvic organs. There are many specific exercises and yoga postures that can be used to relieve common pregnancy discomforts.

Exercise also helps keep you feeling comfortable in your changing pregnant body, and certain forms of exercise, for example, yoga, help you "tune into" your body more deeply. Exercise can help you stay relaxed and get toned at the same time.

Many of us experience resistance to exercise—we find it hard, we're out of shape, we find it tedious, or we have bad associations or experiences with exercise such as inability to lose weight we were struggling to lose or discouraging experiences in PE when we were in school. And many women are so accustomed to being sedentary that they must muster up the will to get moving. But even fifteen minutes a few times a week is better than no exercise at all.

One excellent way to help you overcome resistance to exercise is to refer to it as movement. Find ways that you enjoy moving your body. What feels good to you—dancing, Zumba, Nia, walking, yoga, tai chi, swimming, tennis, aerobics? During my pregnancies, I chose yoga as a gentle form of toning my muscles and learning how to identify and relax those muscles. I learned to enjoy the sensations of my body moving and the feelings of warmth, improved circulation, improved digestion, better sleep, and mental wellness that rewarded my efforts. In addition,

I loved to feel my baby moving as I moved with and around my growing child. For more vigorous exercise, I took brisk walks and often turned on music with a great beat and let loose, dancing (I love a good dance party!). Belly dancing, originally developed as a form of abdominal and pelvic toning for pregnant women, is also an excellent way to exercise prenatally.

In these years of having babies and making movement an enjoyable part of my life, I have really learned to appreciate and enjoy my body, and my strength and endurance have improved dramatically. How you choose to move your body while you are pregnant is less important than that you do so. Dance, play, get lively, and learn to enjoy your body, whatever size and shape or however toned you are!

However, exercise, when taken to the extreme every day, can have deleterious effects during pregnancy. First of all, childbirth requires the ability to release our muscles as much as it does muscle firmness. In fact, women with backgrounds in professional dance or athletics may have a more difficult time giving birth than those women whose muscles are looser and less toned. If conscious awareness of relaxation is not included as part of exercising, then exercise may actually be self-defeating. Intense exercise also uses up precious calories and nutrients, and if these are not replaced, then exercise can actually contribute to undernourishment. Finally, for many women, heavy exercise, particularly aerobics and similar workouts, reflects control issues and a lot of inner tension. Women may be trying to control their shape, stamina, or to prove their strength without taking the time to feel good about who they are. The ability to give birth requires an ability to yield and to let go. While this does not mean giving up the control associated with autonomy, it does mean that you must give up a sense that you can make your body do whatever you want it to do. For example, while exercise is energizing, it cannot provide you with the rejuvenation that you derive from a nap. If you need to rest, don't push your body with a workout, and don't resent your body for its physical needs. You can't exercise away your stress; you have to reduce stress in your life at its source.

Many of us experience our bodies as what we inhabit rather than what we are. Often we don't like our bodies, comparing ourselves to fashion models, whom few of us resemble. Not liking our bodies translates to not liking ourselves. Exercising in an attempt to look like somebody else is psychologically unhealthy; it disturbs your ability to appreciate yourself for your uniqueness. As your breasts, hips, and waist grow during pregnancy, you may judge yourself harshly rather than seeing yourself as a gorgeous, well-nourished pregnant mama—an image of a creation goddess. If you are not feeling positive about yourself, you are less likely to take excellent care of yourself, so do something about that attitude! It might save you a lot of pregnancy and birth problems.

Be sure to balance exertion with periods of relaxation. Swim a couple of laps, then float on your back for ten minutes, then repeat this sequence; ride your stationary bicycle or do your step aerobics, but intersperse this with a few minutes of deep relaxation. Or end your sessions with five to ten minutes of guided visualization (see chapter 8 for details) or deep relaxation in a tub. The activity followed by the rest will help you identify areas of tension in your body that you can then deliberately and progressively release. This is perfect physical preparation for birth. As you move and relax, pay attention to the sensations of the baby moving or being still within you, and notice how this changes as you relax. All of this will better enable you to allow your baby to move easily through your pelvis and into your arms. As you both move and relax, communicate your enjoyment and love to your baby.

Remember, it is possible to hurt yourself, even with gentle forms of movement such as yoga. As your belly grows, your center of balance will change somewhat, and you may find various positions or activities more challenging. There is no need to prove anything to anyone, or to show that pregnancy doesn't slow you down. To some extent, it should! Pregnancy is a time to listen to and honor your body's messages, not ignore them.

## Posture

Posture is rarely discussed as an important component of prenatal health, and this is unfortunate because proper posture can prevent many pregnancy discomforts, such as low back pain, shortness of breath, and indigestion. I also believe that proper posture can reduce the incidence of urinary tract infections due to stasis of urine in the ureters, as these are less likely to be compressed.

Aside from the fact that many Americans already have poor posture with a tendency to hunch their shoulders forward, pregnant women have the added tendency, as pregnancy advances, to allow the lower back to be pulled forward by the weight of the growing belly. This produces the typical swayback of late pregnancy, also known as *lordosis*, which accentuates the waddling gait of late pregnancy, as the legs are displaced by the hip bones being pulled forward.

While it is natural for pregnancy to affect your posture to some extent, you can learn to maintain excellent posture throughout pregnancy simply by practicing.

Good posture, when standing, is as follows: your head is held high, shoulders are held back but not stiffly, lower back does not curve forward but remains relatively straight, tailbone is tucked under so that the tops of your hip bones are not pulled forward, and feet should be slightly apart. When you are walking, you can practice maintaining excellent posture by keeping your tailbone tucked. To keep your pelvis in a position of good posture, use your abdominal muscles to pull it up in the front and use the muscles of your buttocks to pull your tailbone down.

Poor Posture

Good Posture

When you hold yourself up properly, you are lifting your diaphragm and stomach off your belly, allowing more room for breathing and for food in your stomach. You can feel the difference simply by sitting in a chair in a slouched position and then switching to an upright, erect posture. Or if you sit down and feel either out of breath or full in your stomach, try sitting up straight. If you find yourself slouching when you sit, practice sitting taller by pushing your lower back toward the back of the chair (so that you minimize the curve in your back) and let your feet rest squarely on the floor, with your legs dropped slightly apart. If needed, you can put a small pillow behind your lower back and another behind your head and neck. This is especially good if you plan to relax in the chair. Similarly, when you are sitting up and reading in bed, sit upright, using pillows for support to prevent you from slouching.

Whenever possible, sit cross-legged on the floor. This will improve the strength of your back muscles, and you receive the added benefit of exercising your muscles as you get up and down.

When you lie down, use pillows to ensure comfort. For example, if you lie on your side, rest your bent leg on a pillow to prevent the weight of your belly from pulling on your lower back. You can also tuck a small, soft pillow under your belly to lift your belly slightly off the bed. Many women like to place a pillow between their knees when lying on their sides rather than the pillow under their legs. Either way, it is helpful to have plenty of pillows on your bed as pregnancy advances so that you can try a variety of positions. Comfort while you sleep will prevent you from the feelings of irritability, indigestion, and muscle aches that so often accompany a fitful sleep.

# Essential Movements for Pregnant Women

There are many excellent books on prenatal exercise and yoga, so here I will provide you with only ten prenatal exercises. These are the ten movements and poses that I have found to be beneficial to the circulation, pelvis, and digestion. They will help you identify, stretch, tone, and relax the muscles that will be called upon when you give birth. These exercises can be done individually, or as a set. The order given is a logical progression, but not from the easiest to the most difficult. You can decrease the number of repetitions if you are not accustomed to exercising, or increase them for a more vigorous workout. Use the descriptions and pictures together to best understand the movements. Begin slowly, and rest for at least five full minutes when you have completed the movements. After an exercise session, you can follow up with a relaxation technique (see "Relaxation Techniques" in chapter 8).

I enjoy visualizing my baby surrounded with light as I do each exercise. Soothing music in the background also facilitates relaxation and concentration. I find it helpful to begin each session with a few minutes of relaxation, neck rolls, and deep breathing. Always exercise on a firm but soft surface.

## THE STANDING TWIST

1. Stand upright with your feet about 12 inches apart. Extend your arms out to each side.

2. Exhaling, bend forward at the waist so that your upper body is parallel to the floor.

3. Now inhale as you resume the standing position, legs still apart and arms extended. Gently twist to your right, pivoting your right foot slightly.

4. As you exhale, bend forward over your leg, so that your upper body is again parallel to the floor.

5. Inhale and resume the standing position.

6. Repeat steps 1 and 2, again bending to the front.

7. Follow steps 3 and 4, but this time bending to your left.

8. As you inhale, return to center, and repeat step 1.

   Repeat positions 1 through 8 up to ten times.

## THE YOGIC SQUAT

1.  Stand upright, feet about 12 inches apart, knees slightly bent, and raise your arms over your head, with your hands palm to palm and pointed toward the ceiling. Inhale deeply.

2.  On the exhale, begin to lower your head toward the ground, one vertebra at a time, until your hands touch the floor.

2. a        2. b

3.  Let your buttocks drop down toward the ground and, as you inhale, slowly allow your body to assume a squatting position.

3.

4.  Hold this squat for as long as you can. If you are unaccustomed to squatting, begin by holding the position for a count of ten seconds. Eventually you will be able to increase this to several minutes.

If you wish to repeat this exercise more than once, you can reverse the steps until you are again in a standing position with upraised arms, and then begin again with step 1.

## THE BUTTERFLY POSE

1.  Sit upright on the floor, flat on your buttocks.

2.  With your legs bent at the knees and open to the sides, bring the soles of your feet together.

3.  Holding on to your feet with your hands, draw your heels as close to your crotch as possible.

4.  Gently "flutter" your knees up and down, gradually bringing your knees closer to the floor.

5.  Accompany this exercise with gentle inhalations and exhalations.

6.  Maintain this pose for a greater length of time at each session. Draw your feet in further and bring your knees closer to the ground for increasing difficulty.

Optional: You can try to touch your head to your feet for an added stretch to your inner thighs. Do not try to flutter your legs while you do this.

## THE FORWARD BEND WITH VARIATION

1.  Sitting upright on the floor, extend your legs to the sides, keeping them straight. Inhale deeply.

2.  As you exhale, slowly lean forward, bringing your belly and chest as close to the floor in front of you as possible.

3.  On your inhale, sit up straight, maintaining the leg position.

4.  Repeat up to ten times, getting closer to the floor the more you practice, and holding the forward bend longer.

    Optional: You can also alternate bending forward over each individual leg.

## THE CENTAUR

(created by Jeannine Parvati Baker)

1.  Bend one leg under you and stretch the other straight behind you, as in the picture.

2.  Your hands are in front of you as if your palms are pressing flat against an imaginary wall.

3.  Hold this position for up to two minutes; then switch legs.

    Optional: Maintaining the leg positions, twist your torso slowly toward the side of the extended leg, and lean back toward your foot. Switch legs and repeat on the other side.

## THE BRIDGE

1.  Lie flat on your back with your knees raised and your heels flat on the floor.

2.  As you breathe in a relaxed rhythm, grasp your ankles with your hands.

3.  Continue with the relaxed breathing, and slowly lift your buttocks off the floor as if an invisible string were drawing your belly button toward the ceiling.

4.  Hold this position for up to thirty seconds; then lower your buttocks to the floor.

    Repeat up to four times in a row.

## PELVIC ROCK

1.  Get into a hands-and-knees position with your back parallel to the floor.

2.  As you exhale, let your belly drop toward the floor.

3.  Now inhale, arching your back like a cat.

    Repeat this sequence up to twenty times, following a gentle breathing rhythm.

## LEG EXTENSIONS

1.  In a hands-and-knees position, gently lift your left leg backward and upward, letting your foot reach toward the ceiling.

2.  Return your knee to the floor.

    Repeat up to twenty times; then repeat with the right leg.

## LEG LIFTS

1.  Lie on your left side.

2.  Raise your right leg to the ceiling and make gentle circles in the air with your foot.

3.  Lower your leg.

    Repeat up to twenty times; then roll onto your right side and repeat with the opposite leg.

## THE LUMBAR STRETCH

1.  Lie flat on your back, legs extended and arms stretched out to the sides.

2.  Slide your right foot up and bring your knee toward your chest.

3.  Keeping your shoulders flat on the floor, twist your hips until your right knee touches the floor near your left hand.

4. Breathing gently, hold this position for up to thirty seconds.

5. Return to position 1 and repeat on the opposite side.

6. This can be repeated up to three times on each side.

From this last posture you can easily go into a relaxation position, using pillows as necessary to support your legs, belly, head, and neck.

# Pelvic Health

Most women lack an understanding of their pelvic organs and muscles—where they are, what is normal and healthy, even how they look and feel. Yet this awareness can help you prepare yourself for the birth experience as well as enable you to maintain lifelong pelvic health. Few women realize how much birth can be facilitated by the ability to consciously relax the vaginal muscles. In addition, pelvic tone will prevent a host of female problems in later life such as uterine prolapse and urinary incontinence. Sex will be improved, digestion will be healthier, and you are less likely to experience problems such as hemorrhoids. *Our Bodies, Ourselves for the New Century* by the Boston Women's Health Book Collective is perhaps the best resource for understanding your anatomy, and I encourage you to include this book in your personal library as a reference manual.[1]

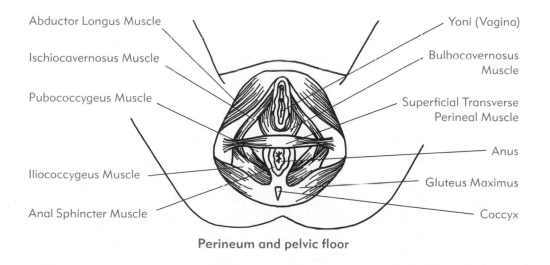

Abductor Longus Muscle

Ischiocavernosus Muscle

Pubococcygeus Muscle

Iliococcygeus Muscle

Anal Sphincter Muscle

Yoni (Vagina)

Bulbocavernosus Muscle

Superficial Transverse Perineal Muscle

Anus

Gluteus Maximus

Coccyx

**Perineum and pelvic floor**

1. Boston Women's Health Collective and Judy Norsigian, *Our Bodies, Ourselves* (New York: Touchstone, 2011).

I will provide a basic idea of the structure of the pelvic bones, the yoni, and the pelvic floor muscles. Refer to the accompanying diagram for visual assistance. The pelvis is a large, bony cradle or bowl that is open at the top and bottom and has various openings within the bony structure allowing for muscles and blood vessels to pass through and attach to the bones: the ileum, the two hip bones that form crests just below your waist on either side of your abdomen; the ischium, which forms the central portion of the hip bones and forms the bones commonly referred to as your "sit bones"; and the pubic bones that meet at the center of your pelvis near your pubic hair line. In the back of the pelvis are the sacrum and the coccyx, also called the tailbone. Your pelvis contains the birth canal, urethra, rectum, bladder, uterus, fallopian tubes, and ovaries. There are ligaments that connect the uterus to the front, back, and sides of the pelvis, and muscles that form a sling beneath the uterus, making up the birth canal and supporting and surrounding this and the other structures. It is these muscles that can be identified and strengthened so that you can work effectively during birth to open your pelvis and also prevent some of the health problems I've already mentioned.

To identify these muscles, collectively referred to as the *pelvic floor*, you must learn to feel comfortable with your sexual organs. Look at anatomy drawings to help you understand what is what and, if you wish (and I highly recommend this), look at yourself in a mirror. You can visually observe yourself tightening and releasing the muscles that surround your external genitals, the same muscles that you would tighten and release to urinate.

## PELVIC FLOOR EXERCISE

Your pelvic floor muscles are best identified as the muscles you use to start and stop your urine flow—although that makes use of just a few of them. Pelvic floor exercises are best known as *Kegels* in honor of the physician who developed them as a treatment for and prevention of urinary incontinence. I prefer to call them pelvic floor exercises. For those of you in a sexual relationship, making love provides a great opportunity for practicing this tightening and releasing, with your partner confirming how tight you can squeeze your muscles during your sexual experience. (Orgasms are natural tighteners of these muscles. They also promote pelvic blood circulation. One mother I worked with referred to orgasms as "assisted Kegels.") Kegel exercises can be done up to one hundred times a day (double that if you've already had problems with incontinence or prolapse).

However, tightening and releasing these muscles is not enough. Women must also learn to tighten the muscles way up in the birth canal in order to gain optimal benefit. This requires some practice, and it can be difficult and even tiring at first. Your midwife can help you to identify these muscles by showing you where they are in your vagina. Or you can feel for yourself. Look in books, or ask your mate to let you know when you are squeezing his fingers or penis. Try to imagine yourself tightening your muscles way up inside behind your pubic bone, not using your thigh or abdominal muscles while you squeeze.

## THE ELEVATOR EXERCISE

Another pelvic exercise is often called the "elevator" by midwives and childbirth educators. The basic imagery is that your yoni is an elevator shaft and you are raising an imaginary elevator from the ground floor (your vaginal opening) to the fourth floor (high inside) using just your muscles. You do this slowly, floor by floor, and then release slowly, floor by floor. You can also release your muscles to the basement by letting them get super relaxed, an excellent practice for totally releasing your muscles to birth your baby when she or he is crowning (head showing and about to be born). The elevator can be done ten times each day in addition to the above exercises.

*One mother I worked with referred to orgasms as "assisted Kegels."*

## HAPPY BIRTHDAY EXERCISE

A final pelvic exercise, one of my favorites, I gleaned from renowned childbirth educator Sheila Kitzinger. In this exercise, you imagine that your vaginal walls are a piece of paper onto which you are writing "Happy Birthday" using your muscles to write. Beginning at the vaginal opening you "write" the H and continue upward tightening and moving your muscles to form all of the letters in these words. You can write any way you want to, but always cross your "t" and dot your "i." Do this ten times each day along with one hundred Kegels for optimal pelvic health.

Note: In order to remember to do the above exercises, choose certain times each day to do them routinely, for example, after each time you urinate, when you wake up and go to sleep, before each meal or snack, or every time you stop at a red light in your car or are at a checkout counter in the grocery store.

## SQUATTING

Squatting is another way to tone your pelvic muscles and is a great position for practicing the exercises described above. Women in traditional cultures worldwide squat daily in order to cook over fires, wash laundry in the river, and so on, naturally promoting pelvic health. The majority of women in traditional cultures are also reported to have had smooth and easy births. Try to squat for ten minutes (or more) each day, building up to it slowly if you've never squatted before. You can squat while you watch TV, play with a toddler, or read a book. Any time that you think of it, squat. Putting a book under each of your heels can help if this position hurts the back of your legs initially. By the end of your pregnancy, you'll be able to squat much more easily, and much to your benefit!

# Massage: Passive Exercise

Traditionally, pregnant women were given extensive massage, often by the midwife, and this was the central component of prenatal care. The pregnant woman might have been massaged weekly or more often throughout pregnancy, with a thorough massage of the belly, hips, and legs. This allowed the mother to be aware of and relaxed in her pelvis, and allowed the midwife to identify the baby's position and massage the baby into the right place if need be. I feel that this physical contact is essential for pregnant women who want to be touched soothingly, especially for women who have a low interest in sex but still want a lot of physical contact. And what adult would turn down a massage? In addition, I am convinced that babies love to be massaged even while in the womb, much as children love it all throughout childhood.

### BENEFITS OF PRENATAL MASSAGE

This healing modality is nearly absent from the care of pregnant women in our culture, and this is a great loss. Prenatal massage has numerous benefits. Being a form of passive exercise, it promotes circulation, which in turn oxygenates the mother's (and baby's) entire body, reducing sluggishness, nausea, fatigue, and depression. It also promotes the release of nutrients stored or stagnant in various parts of the body and helps to relieve congestion of blood, which can result in varicosities and aches.

> WARNING: Varicosities should never be directly massaged as this may release a blood clot, which can result in a dangerous embolism.

Massage gently tones the muscles and helps the mother relax deeply. It can be an excellent sleep promoter for women having sleeping difficulties. It encourages good posture, which in turn prevents both backache and overstretching of the anterior uterine ligaments. But most important, massage helps a woman get in touch with her body. It is an inwardly focused experience that allows her to feel comfortable physically and provides a time and place for identifying and relaxing muscular tension. This is a very important preparation for birth.

Ideally, your partner can massage you throughout the pregnancy, even if it is simply a nightly belly rub or foot massage (the latter being my favorite way to fall asleep late in pregnancy). One needn't be a professional masseuse in order to rub someone firmly and strongly or softly and tenderly, depending upon individual preferences. One only has to be receptive, willing, and sensitive to areas of tension. Massage provides a wonderful opportunity for partners to show their wives how much they appreciate them and is also a ripe time for the dad to feel and talk to the baby. If there is no partner in the picture, another friend can give you a massage periodically—as a gift or as a trade. (Nonpregnant friends would probably appreciate a back rub or foot massage, and this is a nice way for pregnant women to give loving energy, too.) Or you can treat yourself to an occasional professional massage.

Midwives can learn to incorporate massage, taking time to do this in at least a couple of prenatal visits, This can help to develop the feeling of trust and relaxation between you. It also provides an opportunity to teach the pregnant woman's partner how to give her a massage, to identify areas where she may be holding tension, and to help her to release these. It may provide the mother with much-needed touch, especially if she is single or is the mother of young children and is putting out energy all day but has little time to replenish her own.

## GENERAL TIPS ON GIVING A MASSAGE:
## FOR PARTNERS, DOULAS, AND MIDWIVES

Giving an effective massage is really quite simple. The first thing to do is to create a relaxing atmosphere. You will need a dimly lit room that is warm, with a quiet and comfortable spot in which a pregnant woman can relax   plenty of pillows on hand will enable even women in late stages of pregnancy to find a workable position. Soothing music such as the sound of rain or another natural element can help induce a relaxed state.

If the woman will be removing her clothing, then you will need to provide a sheet with which she can cover herself. You will need to expose only small areas at a time, such as an arm, a leg, or her back. This will reduce her feeling of vulnerability and provide her with some warmth.

While it is beyond the scope of this book to offer thorough instructions for massage, I will provide you with a general idea of how to proceed with a full-body massage. Always remember that for a general relaxing massage (in contrast to a specifically remedial massage) your sensitivity, gentleness, and willingness to listen to the mother's needs are all it takes.

Before you begin, remind the mother to use the bathroom, otherwise you can be sure she'll have to get up at some point to pee or she'll be holding onto her muscles, preventing complete relaxation. Then help her to find a comfortable position—lying on her side with one leg over a pillow works well. Now, using a small amount of massage oil, begin by rubbing her feet gently. If the mother wants a firmer and deeper massage you can then press more deeply, but in each area begin gently to allow the muscles to respond and relax to your touch. Work your way up the legs and then proceed to massaging the neck and shoulders. Next, position the mother on her side, if she isn't already, so that you can rub her back. Gently work down her back and over her buttocks. Afterward, you can gently massage the mother's belly, rubbing your hands over it to help her relax her abdominal muscles. If at any time the woman falls asleep, let her rest.

If you wish to massage just one area, such as her feet, simply massage that area more minutely. When massaging the belly, always remember the baby, speak to the baby, and massage her or him, too!

# CHAPTER 8

# The Need for Rest

*One of my very dear friends* would refer to pregnant women as "under heavy construction." I think this explains a lot of why we feel so exhausted so easily in pregnancy—we're working hard building another person! My partner's grandmother, when she was in her late eighties, would always comment whenever she saw one of my babies napping, "Oh, he (or she) is going to grow another inch." She believed that sleeping helps babies grow. There is actually scientific evidence that supports this idea—our metabolism and hormonal levels do differ between waking and sleeping states, and the latter favor bone building and muscle repair!

So cut yourself some slack and make sure you grab plenty of time to rest if you're tired. If you have young children, you are even more likely to be exhausted. Get friends and family members to watch your kids—or hire a high school student to babysit a few late afternoons a week so you can get a nap in or even just some "downtime" to yourself. I like to say that anyone in the family who has the right to brag about the kids should also help take responsibility for them! If you don't allow yourself to rest, you will be more likely to experience fatigue, nausea, indigestion, constipation, lethargy, irritability, emotional swings, and depression. Exhaustion also makes birth and postpartum infinitely more challenging—so practice letting yourself take it easy on a regular basis starting from early on in your pregnancy!

Note that iron deficiency (and other types of) anemia can also make you feel really exhausted in pregnancy. You might also feel short of breath or have other symptoms. Make sure to let your midwife or doctor know about fatigue so that you can get your blood checked for anemia and get appropriate treatment if you are anemic.

# Relaxation Techniques

Taking time to rest does not necessarily mean taking time to relax. Relaxation specifically means letting go of mental stress and physical tensions, at least during the time you are relaxing. You can't make economic difficulties or a leaking roof disappear by relaxing, but you can call a twenty-minute moratorium on worrying, long enough to tune in to who you really are. Since most of us store our anxieties in our muscular, nervous, and skeletal systems, learning to release your worries will help to unlock areas of physical tension as well.

In addition, learning to relax is an essential skill for moving through the birth experience and into parenting with grace and joy. Learning to relax will allow your birth canal to be the path of least resistance. The following exercises are a small sampling of ways to learn to relax. (For deeper stresses and anxieties refer to "Insomnia and Anxiety" in chapter 14, and whenever necessary, seek out supportive listeners or professional counselors.)

- Find a comfortable, quiet place where you'll be uninterrupted. (Remember to turn off the ringer on your phone.)

- Put on quiet, peaceful music to help create a relaxed mood.

- If you have insomnia or find it difficult to relax, try these techniques: first take a warm bath and drink a cup of your favorite relaxing herb tea (a chamomile and lavender combination is excellent).

- If you are a restless type, do yoga or even take a brisk walk. This can help relieve your body of excess energy. Exercise is also a great way to relieve muscular tension, and relaxation is a perfect follow-up to any exercise.

- Empty your bladder before you begin so you're not interrupted by the need to urinate for at least thirty minutes.

Be certain to prop yourself adequately with pillows so that you don't become uncomfortable lying on your back. These exercises can also be done in a chair or lying on your side.

## DEEP BREATHING

Close your eyes and imagine your baby floating or snuggled happily in your pelvis, surrounded by a golden pink glow. Now take a deep breath in through your nose and imagine that breath traveling down through your body to your womb. Let the breath encircle the baby, washing gently over her or him and then let it rise slowly back up through your chest, through your throat, and back out of your nose or your mouth. Repeat this eight or ten times, feeling yourself with each breath being washed over with your baby's love. You can continue to repeat this until you feel deeply rested or until you fall asleep. You can also follow this up with another relaxation practice.

## PROGRESSIVE RELAXATION

Close your eyes and take a few deep breaths, strongly blowing the air out of your mouth after each breath. Continue to take deep, gentle breaths, allowing a slow and gentle exhale after each inhale, as if your breaths are coming and going like waves gently lapping against the seashore.

Now, beginning at your toes, let a warm, tingly, and comfortable feeling spread over each toe. Wiggle your toes slightly, one at a time or all together. Now let that warm feeling spread s-l-o-w-l-y over your feet. Feel all tension and fatigue leaving with your next exhalation . . . .

Work your way over your entire body, continuing from your feet up to your head. (You can also begin at your head and work your way down to your feet.) Relax each area of your body slowly, and deliberately release your muscles as you go along. Imagine your breath as fingers that are massaging away tension in specific spots. Pay extra attention to releasing the muscles in your pelvis, abdomen, and buttocks, areas where women tend to hold tension. Many times you'll find that you've fallen asleep before you get all the way from your feet to your head or vice versa. This is fine and good.

## CREATIVE VISUALIZATION

This process also emphasizes the qualities of using your imagination. Creative visualization, however, focuses on using imagery to induce inner processes for facing and resolving dilemmas, or for imagining yourself how you would like yourself to be. There are many audio tapes now available that have visualizations with lovely music in the background. You can also have someone read a guided visualization to you or tape-record your own. Some excellent visualizations can be found in the books *Transformation through Birth* by Claudia Panuthos, *Silent Knife* by Nancy Cohen and Lois Estner, *Pregnancy as Healing* by Gayle Peterson and Lewis Mehl, and *MotherWit* by Diane Mariechild.

The box below provides an example of a visualization you can do for letting go of anxieties. I was inspired to create this after reading *MotherWit*. To begin, follow the general relaxation instructions and a brief version of the progressive relaxation to bring you into a more deeply receptive state.

---

### Releasing Anxiety: A Creative Visualization

Imagine yourself in a place that is your idea of absolute beauty, security, comfort, and safety. It can be any setting you like—the beach, the mountains, or a cozy chair in a favorite room. This is a place you can return to in your mind whenever you wish to do so.

Here in this space you can safely allow your worries to surface, knowing that they cannot harm you. Now take each image, worry, fear, or anxiety, and, one at a time, watch it grow smaller and smaller. Help it to dissolve before your eyes, let it be washed away by rain or waves, or let the wind whisk it far away. The images are dissolving until they no longer exist. These fears can no longer harm you; they are released from your heart. Feel yourself lighter, relieved of unnecessary burdens.

And now imagine your most cherished ideal for yourself and your family. Whatever it is that you consider nourishing and important, conjure up this vision. Let this vision grow larger and larger. Let yourself be filled with the joy of this image. (Pause for a few minutes until you feel filled with this sensation.)

These positive feelings will grow and develop as you nourish them each day. They are a part of you now and always.

When you are ready, you can return to your regular awareness filled with the joy of nourishing yourself and your baby. Slowly open your eyes, and take a few minutes to breathe deeply before you get up.

---

# Spending Time Outdoors

Spending time outdoors improves our health. It is even better if we can spend time in beautiful places—at a park, the woods, the shore. Walk barefoot; feel the sun on your face and the wind in your hair. Sit on the Earth and feel the pull of gravity drawing you close to her, work in a garden, stroll along the beach, or take a walk in the cool, quiet woods. There is no greater recipe for pregnancy health—for confidence in your body and clarity of mind—than recognizing your relationship with the forces of nature.

Too often women become accustomed to a sedentary daily routine, lived mostly in the confines of houses, offices, cars, stores, and so on, going out primarily when it is necessary to go from one place to the next. This type of lifestyle can cause you to become mentally and emotionally contracted, dwelling on fears, anxieties, stresses, and the mundane details of housework and other responsibilities. While I acknowledge that not all of you who are reading this book will have access to pristine natural settings in which to expand your awareness of the world around you, most women can take a walk in a park, along a river, or near a pond. I myself grew up in an inner city and know that some connection with nature is always possible—even if it's just admiring a tree or the clouds in the sky, or enjoying the purifying sensation of rain on your face. Being close to nature is a reminder that you, too, are a beautiful part of the miracle of life.

# CHAPTER 9

# Physical Changes During Pregnancy

*While every woman is unique* in her pregnancy, there are certain physiological changes that are pretty much universal to pregnant women. The degree to which these changes become uncomfortable, however, can be influenced by nutritional habits, exercise, heredity, available support, and personal outlook. Understanding the changes you are experiencing can help you relate to your body with acceptance and approval, knowing that it is adjusting just as it should.

## Your Breasts

The increasing hormones in your bloodstream can cause breast sensitivity and even extreme tingling or tenderness soon after you conceive and even before you miss your first period. These sensations usually quickly abate, though you may experience heightened sensitivity in your nipples throughout pregnancy and breastfeeding.

As pregnancy advances, women will notice small raised bumps around the areola (the dark area surrounding the nipple). Called Montgomery's tubercles, these are small oil-secreting glands that keep the nipple lubricated. The nipple and areola will also become darker. As pregnancy progresses, some women notice a yellowish or cream-colored discharge coming from their nipples, a wet spot on their bed sheets near their breasts, or a bit of crusted matter in their nipples. This is *colostrum*, the first "milk" that is in the breasts, which will last for the first few days after birth until your real milk comes in. During pregnancy, you will want to look at your nipples to see if they are erect, flat, or inverted. If they become erect in cool air or when you feel sexually aroused, then you are ready for breastfeeding; if they are flat or actually dimple inward even when squeezed or stimulated, then speak with your midwife or a La Leche League leader to learn how to prepare your nipples for nursing. There are simple things that you can do that will enable your baby to latch onto your nipples with greater ease, but these should be done before the birth for an optimal transition to breastfeeding your baby. Flat and inverted nipples need not prevent you from nursing your baby.

Your breast size may increase substantially during pregnancy, which can lead to discomfort, especially if you already had large breasts. If this is the case, a supportive bra in the appropriate size can be helpful, even if you haven't worn one before. You may notice that the veins on your breasts and on your chest are more visible, appearing like the blue lines on a map that mark the location of rivers. As your breasts increase in size and weight, you may notice silvery lines: these are stretch marks.

It is also normal for the breasts to feel slightly lumpy due to enlargement of the alveoli (milk glands). However, it is sensible to feel any lumps carefully to be certain that they are part of normal breast changes. Learning to massage your breasts can be part of a regular practice of loving your breasts and will help you recognize cyclical changes as you become more familiar with your body. In this way, you are likely to notice any problems, should they arise, without the anxiety that a formal breast exam conjures up. Of course, any suspicious lumps should be further palpated by your midwife or other health care practitioner, and, if necessary, further information should be sought to determine the nature of the lump, as pregnancy does not prevent breast cancer (though according to research studies, extended breastfeeding substantially decreases the risk of developing this disease). Remember, however, that most breast lumps are not cancer.

During pregnancy it is important that you be honest with yourself about how you regard your breasts. Many women harbor anxieties, measuring their breasts against cultural standards. If you are unhappy about your breasts, this can hinder breastfeeding. For example, if you have always felt that your breasts are small and inadequate, you may also worry whether you can produce enough milk (small breasts can produce as much milk as large breasts), or if you are embarrassed about your breasts you may hesitate to nurse your baby in public and may feel uncomfortable and inhibited in general. Talking to your midwife or a La Leche League leader can be helpful.

## Your Yoni

Vaginal changes also occur early in pregnancy, with the birth canal becoming a purplish color and the amount of vaginal discharge increasing. The yoni and vulva become quite engorged during pregnancy due to increased blood flow to the area. This can greatly increase sexual sensitivity and pleasure. The increased amount of discharge can cause considerable wetness, to the point of it being completely normal to change your underwear during the day.

Increased wetness can also promote the growth of vaginal organisms such as yeast. This can lead to itching, burning, or irritation, increased need to urinate, and discomfort during lovemaking. Depending upon the type of organism, it can also cause the discharge to become thicker, with a creamy, yellowish or greenish color and an odor ranging from a mild "bread-yeast" smell to a strongly unpleasant fishy odor. (See "Vaginal Infections" in chapter 14 for treatment suggestions.)

In addition to the birth canal and vulva becoming engorged, so does the cervix. It also becomes softer and more likely to bleed if it is touched or scraped. Therefore, it is not uncommon for pregnant women to notice a few spots of blood or pink-tinged vaginal mucus after sex.

## Digestive Tract

Most pregnant women are familiar with the digestive changes that pregnancy brings: an increased sensitivity to smell, a change in food preferences, slower digestion, nausea, indigestion, lack of appetite, and bowel changes. Most of these changes are due to increases of progesterone and estrogen and to the increasing pressure of your growing baby and uterus on your digestive organs. There might be increased sponginess of the gums—hormonal changes cause them to bleed more easily. Pregnant women should take care to brush and floss regularly but gently, and to maintain an excellent diet rich in iron, vitamin C, and bioflavonoids.

To some extent, some of the digestive changes of pregnancy are unavoidable and normal. However, with excellent nutrition and attention to rest and exercise, many prenatal digestive discomforts can be reduced or prevented.

# Urinary Tract

Due to increased blood volume, pressure from your growing womb, hormonal changes, and incorrect posture, pregnant women experience a marked increase in the need to urinate. This can be as frequently as every couple of hours during the first trimester and even more frequently during the last months of the pregnancy. Most women will also need to urinate at least once during the night, but sometimes as often as two or three times in late pregnancy. You may also need to go when you stand after having been sitting for a while, and as soon as you get in the car to go on a long journey! Most pregnant women will notice that they don't urinate quite as frequently during the second trimester. This is because the weight of the uterus has lifted somewhat off the bladder. If you are experiencing extreme urinary frequency, discomfort when you urinate, backache, frequent uterine contractions, or flu-like symptoms, see "Urinary Tract Infections" in chapter 14. It is beneficial to use herbs such as dandelion, nettle, and chamomile regularly, as they promote kidney health, prevent urinary tract infections, and have general nutritive value.

Due to the pressure of the womb on your bladder, you may notice that you occasionally dribble a bit of urine when you sneeze or if you run or jump. This may also be due to weakness of the pelvic floor muscles. It is to your long-term advantage to begin now to strengthen your pelvic muscles to prevent later problems of incontinence or prolapse of your pelvic organs (see "Urinary Incontinence" in chapter 14).

# Uterus and Belly

The most obvious change your body goes through during pregnancy is uterine growth. This transformation is generally very exciting, though at times anxieties may arise. You may wonder how much more you can really stretch, or whether you will ever be able to see your toes without bending over. A pregnant woman's belly receives a great deal of public attention as well, some of it welcome, some unsolicited and unwelcome. Strangers and friends alike rarely fail to comment on how big or small a pregnant woman is, on whether she carries her baby like it's a boy or a girl, and so on. With all of this attention, it is easy to overlook the incredible miracle that your body is manifesting.

The uterus grows from the size of a small pear to a large watermelon. Your womb increases in weight from a couple of ounces to about two pounds. It is an incredible structure capable of growing to such a size and then returning to its pre-pregnant size in a matter of weeks. In addition, it serves the marvelous purpose of sending your baby forth from your body and into the world. The layers of the uterus also have built-in mechanisms for contraction that prevent excessive bleeding after the birth.

Your womb will grow steadily throughout pregnancy, with the baby having occasional periods of more- or less-rapid growth. By about twelve weeks, the top of the uterus, called the *fundus,* can be felt just above the pubic bone, and by twenty weeks the fundus is usually at about the level of your navel. At approximately thirty-six weeks, your uterus will be pushing up against your diaphragm and you'll probably be wondering how much bigger you're going to grow. Then about two weeks before the baby is likely to be born, the baby will drop down slightly into the pelvis. While this gives you more breathing room and room for food, you'll likely be urinating a lot again. For some women who have already given birth, this shift, known as "lightening," may not occur until labor begins.

*It is an honor to become a parent. A mother is the doorway through which we gain entrance into this world.*

—DIANE MARIECHILD

Of course, all of this growing means that your body is doing a lot of stretching and growing around the middle (and everywhere else). Many woman are afraid of putting on weight, fearing that they'll never lose it again. It is true that pregnancy changes our bodies. In general, we become just a little softer and certain changes such as stretch marks are permanent, though they do fade with time. If we can accept the beauty of our bodies as they are, not comparing ourselves to a cultural ideal, and commending ourselves for our incredible ability to bear children, these changes will be accepted and needless tension will dissolve. In fact, if we could redefine the standards of beauty for women's bodies, our whole culture would be healthier and more sane. It is up to women to claim our pregnant bodies as beautiful and powerful. Only by each one of us changing our attitudes can society change its attitudes. We are not meant to be teenagers forever—we are meant to become women, with all of the aging and stretching that goes along with this transformation.

During pregnancy you may notice periodic and irregular tightenings or contractions of your uterus. This is not generally an uncomfortable sensation; you may merely notice that your belly feels very hard for a matter of seconds. These contractions may get more frequent or last longer as you get closer to the time of labor. They are more likely to be noticeable in your second or succeeding pregnancies. You are also likely to notice such contractions after orgasms. These contractions are in fact beneficial as they serve to tone your uterus and help to regulate pelvic blood flow. Only if they become regular, of stronger intensity, or progressively closer together more than three weeks before you are due will there be any need to contact your midwife or health care practitioner to try to stop the contractions.

## Hair and Skin

For most women, pregnancy brings enhanced hair and nail growth, with hair becoming lush and thick for the duration of the pregnancy. I've also heard stories of women's hair changing color during pregnancy, generally becoming darker, though I've never heard any scientific reason for this phenomenon, nor have I seen it. Many women will notice accelerated underarm and pubic hair growth as well. This usually stops after the birth, and in fact much of the new growth may fall out during the first year after birth.

Your skin can also go through a variety of changes during pregnancy, ranging from darkening of the nipples, development of the line of pregnancy that extends over your abdomen, and the mask of pregnancy, a brownish discoloration over the eyes and on the forehead that resembles a mask (and is perhaps a sign of folic acid deficiency), to an increase or a decrease of preexisting skin troubles such as acne or eczema. Itching may also be noticeable, particularly as pregnancy becomes advanced. Whether the problems clear up or are exacerbated depends upon your diet. The healthy functioning of your liver will help to process the hormones that can trigger skin troubles. Healthy bowel and kidney functioning will also help to reduce skin problems as the task of elimination will not rest so heavily on the skin if your other systems are performing their eliminatory functions optimally.

During pregnancy and through the first months after birth, women generally sweat much more than usual and with a stronger odor. This increase in sweat is both due to hormones stimulating the sweat glands and due to the extra heat of pregnancy from increased metabolism and subsequent sweating, a cooling mechanism. Again, a healthy diet with good elimination should reduce strong body odors, and a natural deodorant (one that contains no aluminum, is based on natural ingredients, and is not an antiperspirant) may also help. In her book *Holistic Midwifery*, Anne Frye suggests taking 1 to 2 tablespoons daily of liquid chlorophyll to help reduce body odor and provide extra nutrients at the same time.

# Bones and Muscles

Contrary to popular assumptions, pregnant women do not suffer bone loss or tooth demineralization if they eat a well-balanced diet. In fact, pregnancy enhances calcium uptake, and though some bone loss may occur during lactation, this is replaced when your child stops nursing. Of course, a nourishing diet rich in minerals is essential.

Due to the influence of hormones, in late pregnancy you will notice that your joints, especially in your pelvis, feel looser. You may notice tenderness or outright discomfort or a feeling of mushiness. You may even notice clicking sounds in your pelvis as you walk or roll over in bed. It is this same loosening effect that allows the pelvic bones to separate slightly to accommodate the baby's head. You should pay attention to your posture, as the loosening of the joints and the slight relaxation of the abdominal muscles can lead you to sway your back and consequently develop low-back pain. All of these changes are more likely to register as complaints and discomforts if your muscle tone is already lax, particularly if you've had a number of children already. Regular exercise (both before and during pregnancy) and good posture are beneficial.

# Touch, Sound, and Smell

Sensitivity to touch and sound are generally enhanced during pregnancy (much to the chagrin of mothers with toddlers!) as is the sense of smell. It is very common for pregnant women to be irritated by noise and sensitive to touch.

The sense of smell is greatly exaggerated, though the nasal mucosa may become engorged, leading to a slightly stuffy nose. Taste may be either enhanced or decreased, depending upon the woman, but either way, it is usually noticeably altered. Spatial awareness is also frequently altered—for example, it is not uncommon for a pregnant woman to miss the last step going down a flight of stairs, when her belly prevents her from seeing the step. Her sense of balance may also be affected. Some pregnant women notice that they drop things more easily or that their short-term memory seems fuzzy at times. These are all temporary changes, may not occur at all or only rarely, and may have to do with nutritional needs—for example, anemia may affect mental clarity as less oxygen may be delivered to the brain than is optimal.

# CHAPTER 10

# Emotional Changes by Trimester

*Just as pregnancy changes us physically,* it changes us emotionally. This is a normal and healthy part of becoming a mother, and there seem to be universal emotional themes that run throughout the trimesters of pregnancy. Pregnancy is a time of heightened emotion due to massive amounts of circulating hormones (think PMS times infinity!). And it is a time when we naturally experience a wide range of concerns and anxieties; after all—it's a high-stakes process!

The themes that infuse women's emotional and psychological issues are very similar, often reflecting the specific stage of pregnancy the woman is in at the time.

Stress can have a significant impact on our health, so while some amount of concern about becoming a mother, going through labor and birth, finances, and so on is entirely normal, expected, and par for the course, reining in out-of-control emotions deserves as much attention as a nutrition or exercise plan. Past experiences such as a miscarriage, difficult pregnancy or birth, or problems with a surviving child can all surface as anxieties, as can childhood traumas. Also, depending upon individual circumstances, each of us has our own unique concerns, such as being a single mother, a mother who works outside the home, a mother carrying two or more babies, a woman in a stressful partnership, with financial issues, with sick parents—you name it, and someone is probably struggling with it.

You may feel, as do many pregnant women, that you are the only one experiencing anxiety, ambivalence, fear of birth or motherhood, or sexual tensions with your partner. This is not true—and you do not have to be embarrassed talking about these experiences with your midwife, doctor, or a therapist who specializes in prenatal issues. Getting help is important. Unresolved problems can lead to insomnia, poor eating habits, high blood pressure, rapid pulse, poor weight gain, and many other symptoms. Not addressing these symptoms can lead to complications in your pregnancy or in giving birth. This section is intended to let you know that most women have many anxieties during pregnancy, and that you are definitely not alone or crazy!

# First Trimester

The first trimester is a time of integrating the fact that you are pregnant. For some women who have wanted a child, this will be a joyous realization. For some women, the news will be a surprise. Some women will be outright unhappy to be pregnant, having not planned or wanted a baby at the time.

Some ambivalence is usual in pregnancy and will not cause physical harm to the baby. If you are experiencing ambivalence or if you do not accept the fact that you are pregnant, you can discuss the matter with your midwife or health care provider. Either can guide you in letting your baby know that it is nothing personal, that you have some issues to work through. It may take several months to integrate the pregnancy, particularly if it was unexpected. This ambivalence is generally increased by the nausea, exhaustion, and other physical discomforts common to the first trimester. As these discomforts begin to subside, it is very common for the ambivalence to subside as well. However, it is a good idea to discuss your feelings openly with your partner, midwife, or trusted friend so that you don't overload yourself with worry or guilt.

Feelings of nausea and other physical discomforts can also cause you to feel extremely incompetent and dependent, particularly if the nausea is severe or you have other responsibilities such as children or work that you don't feel capable of doing. This can lead you to feel very discouraged about your ability to cope with pregnancy and to wish it were all over. Being dependent on your mate for extra help can also lead to tension, especially if he does not understand how terrible you feel. If both of you discuss your situation with your support person(s), it can help resolve the tension and get you the support you need without you feeling guilty for needing it.

How a partner responds to the news of your pregnancy can also influence you. You may get angry at him, feel rejected and depressed, or worry whether you may have to bear the child as a single mom. Many women find that during pregnancy, they feel an intense desire to be with their partner practically all of the time to develop a very intimate connection. Unfortunately, men who are feeling anxious about the responsibility of fatherhood or who are not accustomed to such bonding may feel boxed in. Open communication and learning to feel centered are essential skills for a healthy relationship. While it is perfectly reasonable to want the baby's dad to be excited about having a child, many men experience a wide range of complex emotions and may not have the grace to show excitement so that you can feel secure in the situation. Hopefully you will both come to a place where you can joyously support each other in welcoming your child into the world. Nevertheless, you must first learn to feel secure in yourself.

The hormonal changes of pregnancy can cause strong emotional fluctuations and a heightened sensitivity that can lead to unexpected, new emotional outbursts, such as weeping, anger, taking things personally or feeling rejected (particularly with your mate), and sentimentality (such as crying over a children's story or a song on the radio that would never otherwise make you gush). Nausea, fatigue, and hunger can exacerbate some of the more unpleasant outbursts. On the brighter side, you are also likely to experience new levels of elation, sexual union, and joy, and a deep connection to living beings.

The first trimester is often accompanied by a sense of disbelief that you really are pregnant. I can recall that with each of my four pregnancies I would expect to see menstrual blood each time I wiped after urinating. Many women will wait with bated breath for any physical indications of pregnancy, and with each increase or decrease in breast tenderness or nausea will think, "Oh, I really must be pregnant" or "I guess I'm not pregnant after all." Even with a positive pregnancy test, women will wonder if it was a false reading.

If you have a history of miscarriage, you may anxiously wait until you are past the point where the miscarriage occurred in the previous pregnancy. This can be a very stressful time in which you don't allow yourself to become attached to this new little person, afraid that this baby too could be lost to you. However, the actual process of working to connect with your baby, as painful as this may seem, can help you to maintain your pregnancy. Even if the baby is not going to stay with you, a strong spiritual bond can exist for you, and you can help that being on its way. Similarly, a woman may put off bonding with her baby prenatally until she receives the results of prenatal testing (for example, amino or alpha-fetoprotein), which confirms her baby's wellness, rather than loving the child regardless. If you are planning to keep your baby even in the presence of a potential abnormality, there is no reason to avoid developing an emotional bond with your baby prenatally, and for as long as you are gifted to enjoy his or her presence.

## Second Trimester

During midpregnancy, most women will feel at the peak of health and energy. At this point, your belly has become more obvious and your baby begins to move, giving you a very tangible sense of her or his presence. This movement will make the experience finally real for the father as well, enhancing your connection. People, even strangers, may notice that you are pregnant, and you may find it fun to receive the extra attention.

The second trimester, however, is not without its own emotional nuances. General concerns such as finances or other problems may still worry you, and if you are looking after other children, particularly toddlers, you may still feel more tired than you do usually. The middle trimester is often a time of reflecting on your own childhood and on your relationship with your mother. It is perfectly natural for you to need your mother's support during pregnancy, yet at the same time to evaluate what your mom did that you would or would not want to do with your own child. In this generation, many women who want to have natural pregnancies and follow natural birthing and parenting styles may find it difficult to call upon their mothers, as most women in previous generations did not have such experiences and do not know how to talk to us about nutrition, birthing consciously, or breastfeeding our babies. This can lead to you rejecting your mother, and it can prompt tension in a relationship that you want to be nourishing. You also may want your mom to treat you as an adult woman. But because she may give advice or treat you as a child, you may feel unacknowledged in your own transformation into motherhood. All of these feelings may be confusing but in the long run can often bring you closer to your mom. For women who come from seriously abusive families, the complexity of issues may be greater and may have an impact on your pregnancy and parenting experience. It can be helpful to seek the support of an experienced counselor and to discuss such matters with your midwife.

Another common concern that women express during this time is a deep fear that something horrible will happen to their mate, leaving them alone with the baby. In fact, many women have such fears about birthing the baby without the dad that it will bring them to tears. This anxiety can cause these women to worry when their partner is late in arriving home and can also cause them to get angry if he didn't call to let them know he'd be late. If you are economically dependent on your partner, you may worry about how you would support yourself if a tragedy occurred. To reduce your anxiety, you can ask your partner to give you general notice if he won't be at an expected place at an expected time. Clear communication from you can let your partner know how important an issue this is to you.

The second trimester is also a time when women tend to become obsessive about dreams (which may be exceptionally vivid during pregnancy) and about comments people make (which are not always considerate). For example, it is not uncommon for a woman to have a dream that her baby has a deformity, nor is it uncommon for someone to tell a pregnant woman a pregnancy or birth horror story. You may find yourself wondering over and over if a worrisome dream is true or if a person's horror story is some kind of message that this is going to happen to you. While these ruminations are perfectly normal, they don't help you feel positive about your baby or pregnancy; the only purpose they serve is to help you to find your confidence and courage: trust that you are doing your best by consciously caring for yourself and your baby.

## Third Trimester

By late pregnancy, you may be feeling more physically tired again, needing to rest in the afternoon or go to sleep earlier.
If you already have kids, you may find yourself falling asleep while you put them to bed. You probably have to urinate a couple of times at night, and you may find it hard to eat much before you feel full. In general, all of these sensations may propel you to feeling ready to give birth. At the same time, you may feel overwhelmed by preparing your supplies or getting your home ready for the baby. Many women become obsessive about having a clean house, scrubbing areas that are usually overlooked such as the corners of cabinets, the baseboards, or spots on the walls. This seems to be a normal, almost instinctive need at this time. However, it is important that you are able to let go of being compulsive, trusting that you will be ready when the time is right, and that as long as your home is generally clean, the baby doesn't really care how the cabinets or baseboards look.

You may not feel obsessively worried about your mate any longer, but may now worry that you yourself may die while giving birth. This seems to be a particularly

*Happiness, joy, awe, wonder— to think of a baby, a new life growing within—what a miracle. I had some feelings of fear especially when intense nausea and fatigue set in. Just fear like how would I be able to take care of everyone.*

—LISA OLKO, mother and midwife, journal entry

worrisome thought for women who already have children. You may also worry that if you and the baby are okay, something may happen to one of your older children. Such anxieties are perfectly common and reflect how important your family is to you. They may also help you see how much you value your life and your commitment to your baby. We are too often trained to expect the worst or to feel as if we can't have it all, causing us to mistrust the future. This is, again, a time to call upon your trust in yourself that if you've done all you can to be healthy (and likely you have), then you are healthy. It is very rare for women to die in childbirth in affluent countries such as this.

You may also feel depressed about the size of your body, uncomfortable in all of your clothes, and awkward as you engage in physical activities. Physical fatigue may cause those of you who already have children to worry how you will cope with the baby. Remember that you will have hard days and smooth days, and that the better you eat, rest, and refresh yourself emotionally, the better you will cope in the future. Sex may also feel awkward at this stage. You and your mate may need to try different positions so that you feel comfortable. If you honor the beauty of your pregnant body (and take care to exercise regularly to maintain your limberness), you will feel more comfortable in late pregnancy and have a more positive body image.

Toward the end of pregnancy, many women find themselves more "spaced out" than usual. You may find yourself daydreaming about your birth or baby, or preoccupied with other details that you feel the need to attend to before your baby is born. While you are no less capable of dealing with concrete tasks, you may prefer to bask in a warm bath, take a long walk, or write in a journal. It is normal and actually beneficial to take the time to tune in to your more intuited needs at this time. A natural birth is best facilitated when you are able to enter into a relaxed, reflective, and intuitive state.

# CHAPTER 11

# The Month Before Birth

≫≫≫⋘⋘

*During the last four to six weeks of pregnancy,* you may feel eager to prepare yourself for birth and to meet your baby. This anticipation is welcome. You might also be feeling really overwhelmed and anxious about the birth. There's no one right way to feel, and most often we feel a mixture of emotions!

You may also be facing new discomforts now that your belly is so big—you're probably peeing frequently, having difficulty eating much more than a small portion at a time due to less physical space in your stomach; you may be more fatigued, partly because your sleep is interrupted due to difficulty finding a comfortable sleeping position (and getting up to pee!); you might have heartburn, indigestion, and so on. (Definitely try some of the suggestions for addressing common pregnancy discomforts presented in the next part of the book if you haven't been able to fully prevent them with the good tips you've read up until now!)

During these last weeks of your pregnancy, you may have many questions for your midwife or other care provider, especially about birth and caring for babies. There are no silly questions, and since you will be seeing your care provider more regularly, you can use the time to become better informed.

As the end of your pregnancy approaches, you may also begin to wonder whether you can really do it or to feel that you just aren't ready yet. This is a common anxiety, a reckoning with the forces of birth that you are about to face, and an awareness of the great responsibility of parenting. There may also be other anxieties or feelings of ambivalence. The best way to resolve these is to discuss them openly. By admitting worries and asking for help, you are more likely to facilitate your birth. By holding back, you may actually hold the birth back, as your hormones and muscles mirror your emotions. Midwives are usually prepared, willing to listen to your concerns and help you face and work through these feelings. By acknowledging and addressing your doubts, and arriving at a place of confidence before you enter labor, you will be in a stronger state of mind for birth.

How well you care for yourself during late pregnancy can strongly set the tone for your birth experience. This chapter is devoted to helping you continue caring for yourself optimally during these last weeks of pregnancy so that the tone you set is positive. It explores ways that you can prepare your body and nourish your spirit so that when the time comes for your baby to be born, you will be ready, willing, strong, and healthy.

## Nutrition and Rest During Late Pregnancy

A mother who enters labor tired and poorly nourished stands a very great chance of not being able to cope with the intensity of the process, of having a dysfunctional labor in which her uterus does not contract effectively, and of eventually requiring interventions that enable her body to birth or be delivered. Sleep and nutritional deficits are easy to prevent and even cure during pregnancy with adequate emotional support and extra help with daily chores if needed, good nutrition, and appropriate supplements if needed. It is therefore of tremendous importance that you pay close attention to your body's needs during this time.

### SLEEP AND RELAXATION

When you are tired, stress seems magnified and pain is less tolerable. When you are fatigued, emotions seem to take on a life of their own and your body will function less effectively. It is standard for you to tire more easily during late pregnancy than at other times in your life; you are working constantly, even when at rest, to grow your baby. When you ignore your body's need for rest, problems begin to arise. The simple solution is to rest regularly, napping in the afternoon whenever possible and getting to bed early. (I generally recommend that women try to get to bed by 10 p.m. during the last weeks of pregnancy.) These habits will ensure that you will be well rested so that if you begin labor at 2 a.m., for example, you will have had some sleep.

If you are unable to take a regular afternoon nap, a short period of deep relaxation can substitute. Chapter 8 provides several suggestions and techniques for deep relaxation. It can be done before you go to sleep at night, enhancing your sleep. It can't be overstated that you must be well rested during late pregnancy.

Birthing can take a long time, and you will be able to meet this challenge only if you meet your body's needs beforehand. It should be clear that fatigue can actually prolong labor.

## NUTRITION

For most women, late pregnancy brings fluctuations in appetite ranging from being ravenous to not having much appetite at all. Your increased appetite will be in proportion to growth spurts that your baby has in the last weeks of pregnancy. A loss of appetite often occurs at this time because you have a sense of fullness as your growing baby presses against your stomach, leaving much less room for food than you had earlier in the pregnancy. It is important to maintain excellent nutrition throughout your pregnancy, since this will keep you in top preparation for birth, which requires an enormous expenditure of energy. If you find that you are tired of the same old same old, treat yourself to a new recipe book or ask your friends or your midwife for recipe suggestions. Sometimes just having a change of foods can spark your appetite.

As your baby grows and you find it difficult to eat a quantity of food at one sitting, you may want to eat small but frequent meals throughout the day and into the evening, avoiding foods that might contribute to heartburn (tomatoes and peppers are common culprits). It is very important to eat sufficient complex carbohydrates, proteins, and iron-rich foods at the end of pregnancy. The complex carbohydrates will help maintain stable blood sugar levels, keeping your energy levels steady as well. The increased protein and iron are essential, the protein for the rapid development of the baby's brain and the iron for storing in the baby's body for the first six months of life. If you have a consistently poor appetite, anemia may be an underlying cause and should be treated using the recommendations in chapter 14, under "Anemia."

# Herbs for Late Pregnancy and Birth Preparation

Some women and midwives use herbs during the last three or so weeks of pregnancy to "prepare" the body for labor. Such herbs, traditionally called *partus preparators*, were historically used to make labor shorter, less painful, and easier. While this is certainly a set of goals I suspect most pregnant women would love to achieve, I don't recommend the use of partus preparators. First of all, the use of such herbs to prepare women for labor begs the question of why one would use an herbal preparation to ready the body for something it naturally knows how to do? As my grandmother used to say, "If it ain't broke, don't fix it!" Second, not all of the herbs used this way are considered safe.

Classic partus preparators include blue cohosh (*Caulophyllum thalictroides*), black cohosh (*Actaea racemosa, syn. Cimicifuga racemosa*), partridge berry (*Mitchella repens*), and spikenard (*Aralia racemosa*). Blue cohosh is the most notorious, having been written up in three case reports associated with poor outcomes for the baby. While these outcomes were likely due to a combination of factors, of which the blue cohosh was just one and not necessarily causative, the herb does contain chemical compounds that may restrict blood flow to the baby. Therefore it should never be used in late pregnancy, and should only be used by a skilled practitioner if indicated during labor (many midwives use it to help induce labor and to stimulate contractions in labor if they have stalled).

The only herb with proven safety during pregnancy as well as efficacy in facilitating labor is red raspberry leaf (see my "Nourishment Tea" on page 86). Several studies have shown that drinking the tea, even at a dose of 1 to 2 cups per day (I usually recommend 1 tablespoon of dried herb or two teabags per cup for maximal benefit) can slightly shorten the length of labor and reduces the need for interventions at the time of birth, including less need for operative and forceps deliveries and less need for resuscitation of the baby. You can drink it starting in the second or third trimester, and even just drinking 1 to 2 cups of tea daily for the last few weeks of pregnancy is likely to offer some benefit.

## Preparing Your Body for Birth

Your body, unhindered, knows exactly how to give birth. Making sure you are as healthy as possible and taking care of emotional baggage ahead of time puts you in a great place to be ready.

Perineal massage is frequently recommended by midwives and childbirth educators as a way to prepare your vaginal canal for birth. Similar to taking herbs to ensure a "speedy labor," there may be some distrust of a woman's ability to birth implicit in the idea of having to do perineal massage for birth to go more smoothly. The vaginal canal and perineum do not need to be prepped or primed to do their job effectively in labor. There is little proof that perineal massage prior to labor reduces the risk of anything but *insignificant* tears. Reduction of more significant tears has not been demonstrated. The only real advantage of perineal massage is that it may provide you with an opportunity to practice relaxing and opening your vaginal area, and this can be good emotional preparation for birth—particularly if you've had a not-so-great relationship with your vagina.

If you would like to practice perineal massage, your midwife can provide instruction at a prenatal visit. Vaginal massage can be done a few times a week or even daily, using either plain vegetable oil, a mild massage oil, or an oil that is specifically made for perineal massage, sometimes available through mail-order birthing-supply companies. An excellent blend can be made at home following the instructions in appendix A for making an oil. Chamomile, St. John's wort, lavender, and calendula are some herbs that may be included in such an oil. Vitamin E oil also makes an excellent addition since it benefits the skin.

Lovemaking is also an excellent way to prepare your yoni for birth if this is something you enjoy during late pregnancy. You may have to be creative in finding positions in which you are comfortable, but the movements of your pelvis are excellent for toning your uterus and your vaginal muscles. Lovemaking can be creative in other ways, without intercourse, if intercourse is too uncomfortable for you.

As discussed in chapter 7, regular movement during pregnancy in the form of dance, yoga, swimming, walking, or other gentle but strengthening activities helps you become closely attuned to your body. This is essential preparation for an active and positive birth in which you are able to work cooperatively with the birth energy. Late pregnancy may require you to slow down some or to modify your activities, but it is highly beneficial for women to remain physically active even until the last minutes of pregnancy. Physical activity will keep your heart and lungs prepared for the work of labor and will help to keep your blood pressure steady, your circulation excellent, and your stamina and endurance up. However, physical activity is effective only if it continues to be in harmony with your physical needs and your baby's needs. Such exercise should help you get loose and relax and tone your muscles—not push you beyond healthy limits.

# Preparing for Breastfeeding

Breastfeeding provides your baby with both perfect nourishment and the continuity of closeness with which your baby is so familiar. Many women wonder whether they will be able to nurse their babies—whether they will have enough milk, whether they have the right nipples for nursing, and so on. These concerns arise more from internalized cultural messages than reality. Most well-nourished women will have a plentiful supply of milk for their babies. and most women's nipples are just fine for breastfeeding. Occasionally a woman will have flat or inverted nipples, where the nipples do not become erect when stimulated by touch or cold, or they actually dimple inward. Women with flat nipples will usually be able to nurse without any prenatal preparation of their nipples other than massaging the area around the nipple (on the areola, the dark circle around the nipple) to break up any tissue adhesions that might prevent the nipple from protruding. Frequently women will have flat nipples before their first baby is breastfed, but will have erect nipples after having nursed their first child.

If you truly have inverted nipples, consult with your midwife, doctor, or a lactation consultant for information on how to prepare your breasts for nursing. Nipple shields, small plastic cups with a hole in the inner layer, which are worn over the nipples for a period of time each day, exert gentle traction on the nipples, encouraging them to come out before the baby is born. You may also need a bit of extra support with nursing after your baby is born, but even if you have fully inverted nipples, you can nurse successfully—it may just take a bit more determination.

There is no need to "toughen" your nipples by rubbing them vigorously with a towel or any such technique that is sometimes recommended. If milk production is a problem, refer to my book *Natural Health after Birth* for a comprehensive discussion and effective suggestions, and work with an experienced lactation consultant—preferably one who has breastfed babies herself.

## What You Need After the Baby Is Born

While this book is not about postpartum care, there are certain preparations for the days immediately after birth that you need to make during your pregnancy. Late pregnancy is the time to make sure that you have the supplies you will need for your baby as well as the support you will need for caring for yourself, the baby, and the other members of your household while you are recuperating from the birth.

## BABY SUPPLIES

I've never been a big supporter of baby paraphernalia. There is very little equipment that you need for your baby during the first months of life. A car seat is essential, but aside from that, all you really need are cloth diapers and diaper covers, appropriate clothing (you will need very few newborn-size things since most breastfed babies will outgrow these in the first week or so), a baby hat (babies lose a lot of heat when their heads are exposed), a diaper bag, a baby blanket, a few receiving blankets, and a handful of soft washcloths. A sling baby carrier is a useful addition to this list—I love rebozos and used a traditional Mayan one for all of my babies—carrying them in it well into their double-digit months!

Baby stuff is a big business, but most of that stuff is not necessary in the first few months (actually, *most* of it is not necessary at all!)—later on a booster seat, a backpack, and so on, will come into the picture.

## HELP AFTER THE BIRTH

During pregnancy, I have my clients consider who of their friends or relatives might be able to come to their home a few hours after the birth to help prepare a nourishing meal for the couple or the family, to run linens that might have been used at the birth through the washer and dryer, and to look after the other children. This allows both the mother and father the freedom to rest and bask in the presence of their newborn without interruption and ensures that everyone will be well cared for. While, for most women, birth is not a traumatic event (in fact, you may feel very energetic immediately after the birth), it is important that you allow people to cater to you. This is a time for you to allow yourself to be nourished by those who care for you.

If you would prefer not to have company in the immediate hours after birth, you can still prearrange for a friend to leave a meal outside your front door, so that all your mate or midwife has to do is warm it and serve it to you. You can also have meals in the freezer that merely need to be defrosted and heated. You can prepare and freeze these in advance or ask friends and relatives to gift you with meals that can be frozen. One of my clients was given a casserole shower by her friends. Guests brought a dish for the mother to freeze for both her late pregnancy, when she might not have the energy for cooking, and also for after the birth. This was very liberating for the both the mother and her mate, as dinners did not have to be a concern for several weeks after the birth.

If you have older children, particularly if they are under seven years old, you will also want to have someone at home with you at least for the first week after the birth who can tend to their needs. This will help the children feel cared for as well as prevent you from becoming exhausted.

If you are in a situation where you live far from relatives or have just moved to a new town and don't know many people and can't easily arrange for support, you might want to hire a doula, a woman whose profession is to provide postpartum care for mothers. A doula will come to your home for the number of hours that you agree upon and will do the housekeeping, grocery shopping, meal preparation, and laundry. Some will even pick children up from school and bring them home. Most doulas also have basic knowledge about newborn care, breastfeeding, and the needs of new mothers, and can therefore provide valuable emotional support and answer some questions that may arise.

# CHAPTER 12

# Pregnancy as a Rite of Passage

*In many cultures,* including our own (as evidenced by first communions, bar mitzvahs and bat mitzvahs, graduations, weddings, baby showers, and other celebrations), it is important to mark life transitions in tangible ways as rites of passage. The ceremony is a milestone indicating that a person has learned what is necessary or has grown to a stage of development that gives him or her the privilege of entering a new stage. In traditional cultures, rites of passage are used to mark the transition from youth to adult responsibility in a tribe, village, or community. During this time, the initiate must demonstrate her or his ability to withstand or endure certain challenges and will also receive knowledge imparted by elders about the new stage to come.

In our society, little recognition is given to the major transformative nature of pregnancy, which, along with its culmination in the birth of a child, is a lengthy rite of passage into becoming a mother. One can call pregnancy a liminal stage, that is, "a phase of becoming." But often, women becoming mothers are not given special recognition as initiates nor are they taught the skills that can support them to be strong women and capable mothers, which was traditionally imparted via the teachings of elders. But we can change all this by acknowledging the important transformative qualities that pregnancy has in a woman's life.

By viewing pregnancy as a rite of passage, you can take it upon yourself to make the most of the process, looking at the entire pregnancy experience not simply as a means to an end (the birth and the baby) but as a valuable process in and of itself. You can make a firm and courageous attempt to become a powerful woman, learning to trust your body and your innate wisdom. By doing so, you will come to realize that filling and surrounding yourself with the aura of strength and wellness will infuse the baby with these qualities as well.

# An Opportunity for Personal Growth

Pregnancy can give us an opportunity to resolve conflicts from the past that may hinder our sense of empowerment as mothers. A time of heightened emotional sensitivity, it is common for past issues to bubble to the surface—and with motherhood ahead, it's a great time to clear out inner clutter! It is perfectly natural and healthy to expect that, as we walk through the doorway of pregnancy and birth, we will feel fear—we are, after all, facing the unknown. This is inevitably challenging as we grasp the intensity of the birth experience as well as the enormous responsibility of motherhood. And there seem to be benefits in what I refer to as "the work of worrying." I've noticed that women who do some healthy worrying during pregnancy and admit to having fears or anxieties are actually engaged in resolving conflicts. Women who deny—either consciously or unconsciously—that they have fears about birth, the baby, motherhood, their marriage, and so on tend to have a more difficult experience of birth. If you can actively look at a particular concern, prepare or educate yourself about it, and then let it go once you've done what you can to address, resolve, or at least contemplate it, then you are actively working out your fears. It is by addressing such fears or concerns that you can find the inner strength for creative problem solving. For example, if you already have toddlers and find yourself pregnant, you may feel anxiety about how you will handle all these responsibilities. Creative problem solving might include arranging support for a while after the birth, making menus or freezing foods during your pregnancy to have for after the birth, and affirming each day your ability to nurture yourself so that you maintain the energy to care for your family.

You might also choose to relieve bouts of anxiety by writing in a journal, nurturing yourself with tea and a bath by candlelight, crying on your mate's shoulder, or drawing a picture of yourself with images of abundant love being showered down upon you by an imagined loving mother. Such visualizing can help to increase your sense of greater energy and support.

# Self-Empowerment

Empowerment refers to the ability to know what you need and to feel confident about meeting those needs. However, for many women, trained since childhood to be accommodating and passive, this is no simple feat. For a pregnant woman to give herself and her child the best care possible, she must relinquish passivity and empower herself to make choices in her health care.

In the present health care system that denies individuality for the sake of efficiency, predictability, and cost-effectiveness, women must become empowered if we are to receive the care we want for ourselves and our families. To accept treatment that is not truly in our best interest is to allow ourselves to become victims. When one chooses something, this is empowerment; when one allows oneself to be manipulated, coerced, or frightened into accepting something, this is victimization. I always remind my clients that they are the ones in charge of their health care decisions, not the midwife, doctor, or anyone else. Short of an emergency situation, it is your voice and your needs that should determine the care you receive.

So how do you become empowered to make health care choices? Often it takes a difficult experience before a woman is empowered. But you don't have to have an initial experience in which you have felt victimized to bring about such revelation. Determination to trust your body and gradually learning to do so is an excellent place to start. Trusting your inner voice and your intellectual abilities, as well as your social competence, and then speaking up for yourself or following your feelings, are also ways to empowerment. Telling a doctor, for example, that you didn't like a negative comment he or she made about pregnancy, birth, or your body, or asking a neighbor not to tell you negative birthing stories is empowerment. Rather than meekly accepting a negative comment for the sake of being polite or for fear of offending someone, you must protect and care for yourself.

Listening to your body, an important aspect of empowerment, means taking the time to be body centered each day. Because pregnancy brings so many new sensations, this is a ripe time for becoming aware of your body. As you respond more readily to your body's cues, they will become more apparent. In the same way, you will increasingly trust your intuition and common sense. You have to trust that you know what is best for you. You can elicit information, advice, opinions, and support, but then you will have to decide how you feel about things.

Experience too, is empowering. Many women have never had the opportunity to spend time with babies and young children, have never seen a woman breastfeed, and have never changed a diaper. Therefore, many women enter motherhood feeling that they lack the skills necessary to care for their young. While much of mothering is highly intuitive, not all of it is. It does help to spend time around babies. The opportunity to assist another mom with the care of her baby, letting her know that you want to be familiar with the feel of a newborn and to feel comfortable with changing diapers and caring for a child, can raise your level of confidence and your sense of empowerment. Reading books to educate yourself about the basic facts of pregnancy, birth, and parenting can be empowering. Learning infant massage, infant CPR, or other skills, and hearing about other women's positive birth experiences can be empowering as well.

Empowerment is taking an active stand that acknowledges your intrinsic worth as a human being and honors your right to choose whether to say yes or no. It is choosing to replace self-doubt and undermining behaviors with self-loving actions, protective of both you and your family. It is only by each of us actively making self-empowering choices that we will create the attitude in our culture that pregnant women know best what they and their babies need for optimal well-being.

## AFFIRMATIONS FOR NURTURING YOURSELF

Affirmations are a powerful tool for personal transformation. Repeating these messages to yourself is a way to consciously and deliberately create an inner sense of well-being throughout your day: the best times are when you wake, during the course of your day, and before you sleep. By repeating affirmations, you slowly but surely remake your thought processes into those that foster wellness. Affirmations are not used to suppress or deny concerns, but rather to dispel nagging anxieties that do not benefit you. They are useful for dispelling the negative messages we have all internalized—for example, that our bodies are not trustworthy, that our intuitive awareness is inferior to science and technology, that we are unworthy of joy and success, and so on. The following list of affirmations is a sampling of what you might use:

- I am a strong and capable woman.

- My body knows exactly how to nourish my baby.

- I have enough love to share.

- I give myself the right to accept love and nourishment from others.

- My baby is healthy and beautiful.

- I love my pregnant body.

- I will let my labor and birth be its own unique experience.

- I embrace the concept of healthy pain.

- I trust my ability to give birth with strength and power.

If you find yourself countering an affirmation—for example, if you tell yourself, "I am a strong and healthy woman" but a little voice pops into your mind saying,

"No you're not, you're weak"—try to figure out whose voice you have internalized and how that happened. Even if you can't figure it out, you may gain an interesting insight. Don't let such negative messages undermine your efforts. As you persist in the affirmations, you will replace the old, self-defeating messages. Remember, language not only expresses your thoughts, it also shapes your thoughts as well as our culture. Merely by shifting your attention to the positive, without denying your concerns, you can nurture health and enthusiasm.

Because pregnancy is a time of great sensitivity and a portal into a new phase in life, it offers you the opportunity to recognize and release your fullest potential as a woman. This in turn will nurture your confidence as a mother and as an advocate for other pregnant women and other mothers. By holding the intention to be healthy and joyous, and by admitting to and resolving doubts, old beliefs, and negative internal messages, you can grow joyously through this rite of pregnancy, becoming stronger and more powerful in the process.

For further suggestions on honoring pregnancy, see "Celebrating Pregnancy" later in this chapter. For more on the healing and transformative powers of pregnancy, as well as releasing emotional and psychological blockages, I recommend the following books: *Transformation through Birth* by Claudia Panuthos, *Pregnant Feelings* by Rahima Baldwin and Terra Palmarini, *Birthing Normally* by Gayle Peterson, *Silent Knife* by Nancy Cohen and Lois Estner, *Open Season* by Nancy Cohen, and *Pregnancy as Healing* by Gayle Peterson and Lewis Mehl, all listed in the bibliography.

## SPIRITUALITY

Each of us has our own spirituality. For some, this might be the religious experience they have in a synagogue, church, mosque, or sweat lodge. For some, spirituality might be experienced during a walk through a sunlit wood, hearing waves crash against the shore, or listening to the sound of rain. The experience of spirit often connects us to something that includes but is somehow larger than our individual selves. Pregnancy offers you an opportunity to experience a heightened sense of your spirituality because during the precious months of pregnancy, you are an individual yet you are also more than this. It is a period of time during which your connection with something beyond yourself is more apparent than when you are in a nonpregnant state—it is at once physical and transcendental.

The awareness that you are participating in the process of creating life may also enhance your spiritual awareness, as you may find yourself connected to the realm that your baby is in, a realm that is at once physical and at the same time mysterious and unseen. Even ultrasound testing, which makes a baby visible during pregnancy, does not explain the mystery and miracle of the pregnancy process.

You may also experience a heightened awareness of spirituality if you find yourself dreaming about angelic realms, "hearing" your baby talking to you, or experiencing an unexplainable "knowing" of who your baby is and what your baby needs. And you may have other insights about your pregnancy, birth, or child. I find that during my own pregnancies, I have increased experiences of precognition, for example, thinking of an old friend minutes before she phones or I receive a letter from her in the mail. This section discusses ways in which you can develop the spiritual aspects of your life during your pregnancy, and how you might use your spirituality to bring you closer to your intuitive awareness as well as closer to your strength as a woman.

## NOURISHING YOUR "WOMANPLACE"

There is eminent value in taking time regularly throughout your pregnancy to create a sacred space where you take time to honor yourself, other women, family, babies, pregnancy, and birth, and affirm and nourish your great strength as a woman.

Within each of us resides what writer and midwife Nancy Cohen has referred to in *Open Season* as our *womanplace*. This term refers to the part of us that innately knows how to be pregnant, birth, nourish our babies, and live our lives in a creative, empowered, and intuitive way. It is impossible to deny even by scientific standards that we are capable of what can be termed intuition or extrasensory perception. Pregnant women, as do all women, have access to this womanplace for information. But first, each of us must identify and then nourish this place. Depending on the ways that you express yourself creatively, you may identify your womanplace as residing in a distinct area of your body—for example, an artist may identify with her hands, a gardener with her feet planted firmly on the ground, another woman with her heart or womb. To make your womanplace come alive for you, you must nourish and call forth this part of yourself.

You can make this place real within you by actively awakening it through ritual and creative expression. Ritual is simply a time set aside regularly for active attention to your womanplace and for creative expression. How do you like to be nourished with beauty, and what kindles your soul? I enjoy putting on music that makes me dance, and after working up a sweat, I like to feel that creative place strong and alive within me. I also like to sing and drum in a dark room with lit candles or in my garden. I enjoy drawing. Do whatever nourishes your sense of strength and brings you closer to your true self, where you feel a sense of spirit beyond your mundane self and where you feel strongly attuned to your body. It could be a walk in the woods, planting flowers in a garden, making love, or having a water fight with your kids. Visualize your womanplace, even draw what it should look like. Set up a special place in your home, perhaps on the top of a bureau or night table, to remind you of your womanplace. Place objects there that reflect the strength of women and the power and beauty of nature, pregnant women, and mothers. This will serve as a visual reminder of your strength and connectedness with other women and the forces of nature. Nourish that place of creativity and aliveness often, and it will be alive for you when you birth as well as when your kids are little and you need to find your inner resources of energy and patience. By doing so, you also give your children the great gift of energy, as they see your vitality and are supported by you in developing their own place within.

## SUPPORT FROM THE WOMEN'S SPIRITUALITY MOVEMENT

The women's spirituality movement can also help you to move closer to your womanplace. Through the writings of such women as Merlin Stone,[1] Marija Gimbutas,[2] Riane Eisler,[3] Vicki Noble,[4] Anne Kent Rush, Starhawk,[5] Jeannine Parvati Baker,[6] Elizabeth Davis,[7] and many others, and through our own spiritual practices and social commitments, we reawaken to the divinity and strength of women. Ancient traditions reveal that long before written history, female deities were recognized and revered as much as "God the Father" is now. To reclaim the self-respect we deserve for our varied roles and talents as both nurturers and women of social power is incredibly revitalizing. Similarly, awareness of women's great contributions to political and environmental change also gives us a sense of collective strength, pride, and power. We come to realize that spirituality, politics, and women's status are all intimately connected to the environment we create for pregnancy, birth, and motherhood, and that, in reclaiming our strength and

1. Merlin Stone, *When God Was a Woman* (New York: Harcourt Brace Jovanovich, 1978).

2. Marija Gimbutas, *The Living Goddesses, ed. Miriam Robbins Dexter* (Berkeley: University of California Press, 2001).

3. Riane Eisler, *The Chalice and the Blade: Our History, Our Future* (Cambridge, MA: Harper & Row, 1988).

4. Vicki Noble, *Shakti Woman: Feeling Our Fire, Healing Our World – The New Female Shamanism* (San Francisco: HarperSanFrancisco, 1991).

5. Starhawk, *The Spiral Dance: A Rebirth of the Ancient Religion of the Goddess: 20th Anniversary Edition* (San Francisco: HarperSanFrancisco: 1999).

6. Jeannine Parvati Baker and Frederick Baker, *Conscious Conception: Elemental Journey through the Labyrinth of Sexuality* (Monroe, UT: Freestone Pub. Co., 1986).

7. Elizabeth Davis, *Heart and Hands: A Midwife's Guide to Pregnancy and Birth* (Berkeley: Celestial Arts, 2004).

wisdom, we can make this world a healthier place in which to live, birth, and raise children.

A particular mother had developed a sacred time of connection with her baby and, very late in her pregnancy (over a week past her due date), had the distinct feeling that her baby was going to be born in the caul, that is, with its water bag still intact around the baby. I told her that some cultures consider this an auspicious sign, and that it is certainly possible, though very rare. That night she began labor, and a few hours later she gave birth to her daughter—in the caul as she'd predicted!

# Celebrating Pregnancy

Pregnancy provides a wonderful opportunity to celebrate not only the coming of your baby, but the transformation of your own life as well. In our country, the traditional form of celebration is to give the mother a shower shortly before the baby is due, passing on to her positive stories of birth and motherhood, as well as giving her everything she needs (and sometimes doesn't need) for the baby. While this ritual has the potential to be a time to disseminate valuable information as well as to encourage and empower a woman about to cross through the doorway that is birth, it is often less relevant, though still a memorable occasion. In addition to this celebration, or in lieu of it, I'd like to share with you the tradition called the Blessingway. I also want to share an enjoyable activity—making a belly mask—that results in a terrific conversation piece as well as a long-lasting objet d'art that tangibly honors your pregnancy experience.

*In my life the physical acts of birthing have been an incredible means for sourcing my power.*

—DIANE MARIECHILD

## THE BLESSINGWAY

The term *Blessingway* derives from the *Diné* (Navajo) culture and language, but such rituals are germane to peoples all over the world. This ritual, taught to me by my mentor, Jeannine Parvati Baker, has become popular among midwives across North America as we have sought to reclaim and create meaningful rituals and beautiful celebrations for our life cycles. Since writing this book nearly two decades ago, beautiful books on the art of Blessingway have been published and can give you more ideas for creating your own. What you'll read below is one of the original contemporary Blessingway pieces to be published and is based on the ceremonies I offered to my own midwifery clients during those early years of my practice.

The Blessingway is a ritual that can be done to honor, celebrate, direct, and emphasize any significant life changes that are occurring, such as a new job, a move, a marriage, a graduation, the onset of the first menses, menopause, a birthday, and so on. While it is a celebration, it is not a party; it is a ritual, a time of focus and concentration on the subject(s) for whom the ritual is being created, and a time to give birth in an atmosphere that reflects the purpose of the ceremony.

The Blessingway has three basic parts: the opening, body, and completion of the ritual. While there are certain elements that are commonly included, they are not fixed. You can create your own ceremony using original ideas or those you glean from other sources. There are several useful books in the bibliography and many others to be found in bookstores. Singing is an important and uplifting aspect of the Blessingway. Look for CDs and tapes at women's bookstores. There are many beautiful recordings of chants, spiritual songs, and even songs for ceremonies and rituals. Many of these songs are quite simple and have repetitions that make it easy to follow along in a large group, even if people haven't heard them before.

The Blessingway does not need to follow any specific faith tradition. You can infuse the ritual with your own religion, but if you are not part of any organized religion you can extract elements from a variety of cultures and religions or create a nature-centered ritual.

A Blessingway can be given by a close friend, a relative, or your midwife, or it can be done by yourself or with your mate and children. It is usually done in the weeks just prior to your due time. Blessingway guests should include only those people with whom you are very close and with whom you feel positive and comfortable. Blessingways can be women only, women only except for your mate, or mixed. A small group is better with Blessingways, as it is easier to remain focused.

Supplies for a Blessingway vary, but the main ingredients are objects that symbolize pregnancy, life, babies, relationships, the powers of nature and Earth, and so on, which can be used to create an altar or centerpiece for the gathering. Guests can bring gifts to decorate the altar. Additionally, there should be lit candles, flowers, comfortable seating (lots of floor pillows and soft chairs), and a special area arranged for the guest of honor, the mother. To the Blessingway, each guest should bring a small gift for the mother, preferably homemade, or of simple and natural materials if purchased. This gift can be a poem that is appropriate, a new hairbrush or hair clip so that she has something new and personal for herself after the baby is born, a gift for the baby, or even the promise of several meals or help with older children just before or after the new baby is born. Each guest should also bring a dish to contribute to a potluck meal or snack after the ritual. Ideally, one person will get a list from the mom as to whom she wants at her Blessingway, and this person will then call the guests and tell them what to bring. The Blessingway should not cause extra work for the pregnant woman unless, of course, you are planning the Blessingway yourself.

Before you begin the Blessingway, create an atmosphere in the area that invites peace, contemplation, and comfort. You are creating a sacred space. Let people know exactly when you will begin, as latecomers can disrupt the energy of the ritual once it gets going. I find that Blessingways done indoors are facilitated by semidarkness and candlelight. Blessingways held outside are quite beautiful as well.

### Opening the Ritual

Opening the Blessingway involves several aspects or actions on the part of the person facilitating the ritual: welcoming everyone and explaining what the ritual is about and why you are doing it. You needn't be historically accurate; simply explain your intention to create a meaningful way of honoring and supporting—Blessing the Way—of your friend who is about to give birth. (If you are doing this ritual by yourself or with your mate, you may wish to mention your intentions for this ritual rather than the explanation.) This explanation can also help anyone unfamiliar with the idea of ritual, who may associate it with horror movies or something scary. Let folks know that the Blessingway is a participatory event, that you are just helping to keep it focused on the purpose of blessing the mother.

Next comes a purification. I prefer the technique known as smudging. I use smoke to ritually remove any energy, thoughts, or feelings that may be negatively influencing any of the guests or the mother, and to welcome in positive and loving energy. To smudge, you light the herbs cedar and sage and allow the smoke to circulate around each person by holding the lit herbs near their body (use a bowl or a large shell to contain the sparks and ashes). You can blow on the herbs to direct the smoke around the person's body. A nice way to smudge is to have each person smudge the person to their left, going clockwise around a circle. If you know other purification techniques, you can substitute your own methods.

Finally, the invocation is spoken, that is, a prayer to invite and welcome all of those spiritual forces (use your own terms: angels of birth, spirit guides, your own higher powers, forces of nature, Great Mother, Heavenly Father, God, whatever your belief system holds for you) that will assist this mother on her path. The tone should be reverent, the room receptive to these spiritual allies, and the prayer slow and eloquent.

This invocation can be given by the person organizing the ritual or someone else in the group. During the smudging or purification, songs can be sung.

### The Body of the Ritual

This part of the ritual is focused on nurturing the mother, encouraging her sense of support and empowerment, and creating a collective positive intention for her safe and joyous experience of birth. It is a time when guests can share their love individually and as a group for the mother and baby. These are the steps that I usually follow when giving a Blessingway. They are open to your own creative input.

Note: After each step in the ritual, it is pleasant to punctuate the celebration with singing. My friend Lisa Olko created handwritten lyrics sheets almost ten years ago that I continue to use at Blessingways. You can write your own by jotting down the words to several songs that you might want to sing. Then photocopy enough pages to hand out to the guests so that each person can follow along. Hand drums, rattles, and other simple percussion instruments can help set the tempo for the music. These are easy to play and add richness to the singing. You can ask guests to bring instruments if they have any. In fact, when I plan a Blessingway, I call each guest about a week before the gathering and let them know that they can contribute to the ritual by bringing items for the altar, flowers, and a verse, poem, song, or thought to share.

Going around the circle clockwise, each guest introduces herself and tells why she came and what she would like to contribute to this ritual. Each person should have the opportunity to place something special on the altar should she so desire.

*As for remedies, yes, the herbs are powerful healers in and of themselves, but healing is deeper and more than the plant. Healing is will and intention—the strong desire for life.*

The person facilitating the group can lead the guests in a guided visualization, perhaps of imagining giving birth as they would wish it to be. Begin the visualization with a deep relaxation exercise so that everyone has the opportunity to relax and benefit from the ritual. (*MotherWit* by Diane Mariechild is an excellent book filled with relaxation and visualization exercises that can be adapted for rituals.)

Give everyone the chance to return to a sitting position in the circle and introduce the idea of grooming the mother. This involves massaging the mother's feet in a foot bath, brushing her hair, and generally doting on her. Utmost sensitivity to the mother's needs and sense of personal space is essential. For the foot bath, use a rectangular bucket wide enough for her feet and with enough water to reach her ankles. Add herbal oils to scent the water and float a handful of herbal potpourri in the bucket, or prepare a strong herbal infusion and let her soak her feet in this. Lavender, rose petals, calendula, mint, lemon balm, and other aromatic herbs are wonderful. While her feet are soaking and massaged by two of the guests, a third person, perhaps the mother's closest friend, sister, or mother, will brush the pregnant woman's hair (sprinkle a few drops of lavender or rose oil on the brush for added effect) and then style it using hair clips, ribbons, and so on. This is symbolic of preparing her "head space" to be ready for birth and mothering. A flower garland, easily homemade with a bouquet of flowers and wire, makes a perfect crown after her hair is completely groomed. I also have a special Blessingway gown that was a gift to me, that each mother dons at the beginning of the grooming part of the ritual. After each Blessingway, it is washed and put away until the next Blessingway.

After the hair is done and the feet massaged, the two women at her feet rub cornmeal over the woman's feet rather than drying them with a towel. This gives the feet a nice glow and symbolizes wishes of luck, protection, and prosperity for the mother as she walks along her path.

When the grooming is complete and all of the grooming supplies set aside, the next step is the Giveaway, when each guest has the opportunity to address the mother. I like to go around the circle clockwise once more and have each guest say something special and positive that she remembers from her own experience of giving birth. If she has never given birth, she can relate some other special experience. Each person will then present her gift, either reading a poem she may have brought or explaining the gift. This is often a teary experience, so give plenty of time for each person to speak. However, if anyone starts getting negative or goes on and on, you may have to graciously move the energy along.

Another lovely thing to do, taught to me by midwife Diane Bartlett (Whapio), is to create a basket of good wishes, decorated with colorful ribbons. Have some strips of ribbon available for decorating the basket. Give each person a slip of paper and a pen and have each write a prayer, wish, or blessing for the mother and baby on her paper; then pass around a small basket. All wishes should be for the highest good of the mother and baby. Tell each guest to read her wish aloud in turn and, as she does, put the paper in the basket and attach ribbons to the basket. When this is completed, you will have a beautifully decorated wish basket that the mom can look at for inspiration whenever she desires. It will also be a beautiful keepsake for the baby. The actual gift giving can be done when the basket has been completed.

### Completing the Ritual

To complete the ritual, the facilitator can ask if anyone has anything further to share. It is nice if all of the guests hold hands and sing. Although I don't know who wrote it, a very special song that was taught to me is this:

> Dear ones, Dear ones,
> Can I tell you how I feel?
> You have given me such treasures,
> I love you so.

*This is sung to the tune of "Soul Cakes," a familiar old folk song.*

Once done, thank all of the participants, most especially all of the helping angels and other beneficent beings who have blessed the mother's way. Welcome everyone to join in a feast and celebration. You have completed the Blessingway ritual.

## MAKING A BELLY MASK

This simple, inexpensive project is the creation of an actual plaster cast of your belly, best done in late pregnancy for full effect. It is made with the same techniques and materials you use for making plaster face masks. Here's how to do it:

1. Purchase about three rolls of plaster gauze at a local craft store. This is plaster-impregnated gauze used for making face masks. You will also need a small jar of Vaseline, an old plastic bucket, and a few rags.

2. Because it is a messy project, it is best done either outdoors where the rain or a garden hose can wash away the drips of plaster or indoors on a drop cloth or inexpensive shower curtain liner. It is preferable to have someone help you with the process.

3. To begin, assemble all of your supplies and fill the bucket with warm water. Take your clothes off (you can leave a bra or short tank top on) and stand on the plastic or drop cloth. Measuring horizontally across the areas to be covered, cut strips of the gauze in pieces long enough to cover your belly (and torso if your want to include your breasts), and additional gauze to add two to three layers of thickness.

*waters rising*
*moon filling me*
*this vessels holds firm*
*but is ready to*
*overflow at any time.*
*so ready for my baby*
*to be born*

4. Now smear a thin layer of Vaseline onto the areas that you will be plastering. This will prevent the materials from sticking to you or hurting when you pull them off. You don't need to smear Vaseline onto your pubic hair—the plaster doesn't stick well to hair. Then, following the directions on the package of gauze, dip the strips into the warm water and begin applying them to your belly. The general idea is to make overlapping horizontal layers leaving no places uncovered and continuing until you achieve the shape of the belly that you want. When you are finished applying the strips, allow the cast to dry for about five minutes; then remove it from your belly, smooth out the edges by folding them back a bit, and put in a dry, protected spot to harden completely. It will take about twenty-four hours to be dry enough to paint.

Paint with acrylic paints, and have someone spray or paint it with a lacquer or glaze for extra protection. If you must spray it yourself, do so only in a well-ventilated area, preferably outdoors.

# CHAPTER 13

# Your Changing Family

><<

*Babies change our lives.* There's pretty much no getting around it! It's a wonderful thing, but it can also be overwhelming!

Whether this is your first baby or your sixth, each pregnancy and baby brings changes to the family structure as you and your mate adjust to your changing needs and the needs of other family members. Older children may be delighted or they may groan, the youngest has to adjust to the idea of a sibling, and your family budget has to stretch just a little bit more. Approached with a healthy awareness of the stresses involved, the changes of pregnancy need not be overwhelming.

Pregnancy can be a joyous time of celebration, anticipation, and integration of this new being into your life. It's also an important time to adjust our expectations of ourselves—as well as learn to ask for and accept help—so that we can realistically accomplish everything we need to in our busy lives!

## Your Relationship with Your Mate

Growing up and in school, we are not typically taught "Communication Skills 101" or "Relationship Skills for Dummies," and we therefore all too often go bumbling through many of our relationships learning by trial and error (often with some hurt feelings along the way—our own and others').

Regardless of how long a couple has been together, pregnancy and a baby change your roles, expectations, and needs. Women who have careers and who now choose to be home as well as women who have never had a job outside the home may begin to feel dependent upon their mates and lose their sense of competence and value, both so important in the transition to motherhood. These feelings may cause a woman to act more childlike or cling to her partner who may, as a result, begin to withdraw. Pregnancy can bring up really complex relationship dynamics. Understanding these can help you both to address them and adjust your expectations and actions.

## COMMON SOURCES OF TENSION

Pregnancy causes parents to feel new concerns and pressures as well as to reevaluate their needs and expectations for support, so this can be a time of stress. In addition, parents may begin to discuss how to raise the child and may disagree, for example, about parenting styles, religion, how and where to birth, whom to choose as a care provider, and so on.

A common source of tension for pregnant couples is how the pregnant woman's physical and emotional needs should be met. For example, when a woman feels consumed by nausea in the first trimester, she may feel too ill to keep up with the responsibilities she typically attends to and may want her mate to help out more. An already busy partner might feel overwhelmed and overburdened by the extra work—and tensions arise. Again, talking and getting help, either around the house or in a relationship counseling environment can nip in the bud what can turn into long-term problems as the family grows and work and home responsibilities increase.

As a pregnant woman's body grows and changes, she may feel insecure about her appearance and may look to her partner for reassurance. While it is important for a woman to like her own body regardless of another's opinion, her mate's attraction to or rejection of her will influence her sense of self. If a woman perceives that her mate is rejecting her pregnant body, or if she or he actually is, this can be a very painful situation. It seems to me very sad that any partner wouldn't find his (or her, as the case may be) pregnant mate beautiful; however, this issue often arises for couples. For men, a common confusion is differentiating between his partner as a lover and a mother—and it may require him to evolve into new ways of seeing his sexual partner. Usually, a frank discussion facilitated by a counselor or a midwife will clear the air and resolve these issues.

Sexual needs are also a common source of stress. A pregnant woman may not feel like having sex during the first couple of months, if she is extremely nauseated or fatigued, or very late in the pregnancy. If suddenly she isn't interested in intimacy, her partner may take this as rejection. Other pregnant women may feel like having sex more often than ever. If your partner's libido doesn't match up, you might mistakenly perceive this as a rejection of you or your pregnant body. If either partner is afraid to hurt the baby or feels embarrassed making love "with the baby there," this can create sexual tension. A useful and classic book is *Making Love During Pregnancy* by Elizabeth Bing and Libby Colman. For ideas on creative relationships as well as intimacy, see *The Couple's Comfort Book* by Jennifer Louden.

## HEALING TENSIONS

If you are both committed to being together, you can learn skills that will enable you to integrate your differences and transcend the difficulties in order to create a vital, dynamic, committed loving relationship. Jennifer Louden's book contains many creative ideas for improving communication, rejuvenating a relationship, and enhancing intimacy both sexually and in general.

The foundation of any marriage has to be two strong individuals who agree to be together because they love each other and enjoy each other's company. Each of you must work on your own ability to be loving, compassionate, strong, caring, and sensitive. Then you can give love because you want to, without your entire sense of self resting upon your partner's response. However, a healthy marriage must be mutually satisfying; if the responses you receive do not nurture you, this will not be a mutually happy situation.

A couple must be able to communicate needs and expectations openly and truthfully. Both partners must feel free to express themselves and must be able to listen to the other with the heart. It is not fair to resent someone for not meeting expectations that have not been expressed. You cannot expect someone to read your mind, a common mistake that pregnant women make when they want their mates to anticipate their needs. It is fair, however, to expect your partner to see your needs as important, since you are carrying this child for both of you. How one expresses needs can also have an impact on whether they are heard. "Love, would you please rub my back" sounds vastly different than "Why don't you ever offer me a back rub? You know I'm tired!" While an empathetic partner might respond lovingly to either message, the first is certainly more likely to elicit the desired response. Again, expressing messages clearly and from your loving heart is essential, especially if you want to be heard by a loving heart. "A Partner's Point of View," later in this chapter, provides further insights on the importance of the father's (or mate's) role in the relationship during pregnancy and should be read by both of you.

Of course, not all marriages work out. In fact, about 40 percent don't. Sometimes we can prevent this by working on a relationship—including getting help from a skilled counselor. Sometimes, in spite of hopes, plans, and efforts—the reality is we're not in a good match and one, the other, or both need out. This is a really challenging time to go through such a major separation, but there is a lot of support for being a single mom, and you can and will find the strength to be a great mom on your own!

## Single Mommas

Hats off to the single moms! It's no easy road. I was raised by a single mom, and since 40 percent of marriages end in divorce (sorry, not to be a pessimist here if you are married—just reality . . .), it's important for you to know right here and now that pretty much all of the data in the world shows that kids raised by single moms do just fine as do kids who have come through a divorce (reality check—first African American President of the United States? Yup, raised by a single mom!). If you are pregnant and single, this is a great time to enlist a really great friend to be "your person" during pregnancy—someone you can count on through thick and thin to help you out. If you're close with your family, let them help you out. Connect with other single moms *before* you have your baby so you can be a support team for each other *after* babies are born. What about sex during pregnancy? Play it really safe and find ways to satisfy yourself, and if you do partner up with someone, make sure you have safe sex; remaining disease free, including from herpes—even cold sores—is critical in pregnancy because, while something you get may be mild, it could be very serious and dangerous for your baby. And you definitely don't want to pick up something more serious yourself during pregnancy whether it's chlamydia, gonorrhea, herpes, hepatitis, or HIV.

## When You Already Have Children

Pregnancy the first time around is quite a different experience than when you have other children to care for. Most first-time moms do not have the same amount of household work and demands that a mother who already has children may face. If you already have children, particularly if they are young, you are apt to be more tired than when you were having your first baby. Yet so many women seem to forget this simple truth and berate themselves for falling asleep at eight o'clock when their four-year-old goes to bed, letting housework slide a bit more than usual, or eating peanut butter and jelly for lunch instead of a high-protein meal with a fresh green salad.

I am writing this section to simply remind you of the importance of taking good care of yourself. It is important to learn to ask for help and to be easy on yourself. Do let your toddler watch an afternoon movie so that you can take a nap. Let your husband help you prepare meals, and enlist older kids in getting household chores done. While A. B. & J. (that's almond butter and jelly!) sandwiches are okay once in a while, by all means don't skimp on your meals. Fatigue can be reduced by eating well and getting plenty of rest, but if you try to be a supermom, you'll probably be exhausted no matter what you do, and your pregnancy and birth may be more difficult for you. Learn to set limits without feeling guilty, and trust that you are a good mom and deserve time to nourish yourself and the baby.

## INVOLVING SIBLINGS IN THE PREGNANCY

I can barely describe the magic and wonder on a child's face when she or he sees a newborn sibling for the first time. Attending births, this is one of my favorite moments. Yet not all siblings react with keen interest when they meet a new brother or sister. Much resistance can be prevented and even melted away by integrating and welcoming children into the life of the baby before it is born.

Only you can decide when you feel it is the best time to tell older children that you are pregnant. I told mine pretty early on with each pregnancy. Should a miscarriage occur, you can explain this to your children gently in a nonthreatening and age-appropriate way.

When children are involved in the pregnancy from the beginning, they tend to marvel with you at the changes in your belly, the kicks and rolls of the baby in your womb, and the sound of your baby's heartbeat. Children will usually, if not either pushed with the idea or protected from it, develop a healthy anticipation and eagerness to meet the little person inside of you and will identify with being a big brother or sister well before the birth, if old enough to understand the concept.

A lengthy discussion about having siblings present at the birth is beyond the scope of this book, but if you plan to have your child attend the birth, there is no finer preparation than being included in the prenatal care, becoming familiar with your birth attendants, and being exposed to your naked pregnant body. If you view pregnancy as a normal fact of life, so too will your children, and if you extend this view to the birth, your child will do the same.

It is empowering to young children to feel that they are capable people and important members of your household. You can ask your toddler to help you prepare a meal for you both and let him or her know that this feeds the baby as well. You can ask your older child to watch a toddler for an hour while you rest or stretch, or you can invite your children to stretch along with you. You can teach them with books and videos about how the baby lives in your "belly." You can ask your midwife or physician to help the children feel the baby's head, feet, or bottom when she palpates your belly at prenatal visits. Of course, if your child is shy about this, she or he should not be forced to participate. If you have been open with your older children all along, they are likely to want to be involved, and most toddlers love to be in on the action.

When children attend prenatal visits with their parents, I always invite them to feel and listen to the baby. I've even done a mock prenatal on little ones who insist that they are also pregnant. I've had little ones hug me when I've left their homes after a sibling has been born, and thank me without being prompted for helping their mommy with the birth. This always moves me to tears. And as I watch the closeness of these children with their younger siblings, I am reminded of the value of welcoming siblings into the process of pregnancy.

## A Partner's Point of View

### BY TRACY ROMM

*A woman's experience of pregnancy can be enhanced by the participation of a loving support person, whether this be her mate or another close friend. This section was written by my partner, Tracy Romm, with whom I have our four kids. He offers ideas on how to support your pregnant partner, how to meet your own needs, and how to honor your changing role as you become a parent. It was written from a man's perspective on becoming a dad, so I've taken poetic license in revising some of the pronouns a bit. —A. J. R.*

Pregnancy and birth present partners with a powerful opportunity to cultivate nurturing qualities and to bond in deep and lasting ways with our mates and children. That active support is optimal for maternal, child, and overall family health has been amply documented in the research literature. Nowadays, childbirth educators routinely expect partners to attend classes, and most childbirth preparation systems assign to partners a key role at birth. All signs point to a shift in the way partner's perceive their place in the childbearing cycle.

Yet how ill-prepared so many of us are. I remember all too well the dominant images of fathers in my formative years. One of the Desi Arnaz and Lucille Ball shows depicted an almost hysterical Desi trying desperately to cater to the every need of an almost equally hysterical Lucy—to the point of an all-hours search for the proverbial pickles and ice cream. Yet where did it get him? At the birth, he became the stereotypical figure of the pacing father in a cramped waiting room, pockets full of cigars, grasping for any word from any white-clothed figure with authority.

There are reasons to wonder whether our current Hollywood models are any better prepared to show us the way. The movie *Nine Months* featured a successful psychologist who took almost the full term of his mate's pregnancy to willingly make a commitment to mother and child. In the end, it required the video image of an ultrasound to win him over, convincing him that the fetus was a child worth loving and working for. In the end, however, he was reduced to a bumbling idiot as he rushed his wife to the hospital, culminating in an adrenaline-induced brawl with another expectant father in the delivery room at the very moment his wife gave birth. At least we men have made it to the birthing chamber!

This section acknowledges the unique and important role for partners in pregnancy. When all is said and done, we are usually the single most significant other in the life of our mates. As they grow this baby, they look to us for many types of support—emotional and spiritual no less than material. Pregnancy is a dance, admittedly a new one for many of us, and it often takes a while to learn the steps. Take heart. To paraphrase an African proverb, if you can walk, you can dance; if you can talk, you can sing.

## BECOMING A FATHER

When Aviva and I confirmed the conception of our first child, I was truly exhilarated. I felt as if I were walking on air—literally. All of the pressing concerns of my life seemed to melt away in the rosy glow of those first days. Perhaps I

*The path of the mother should be given its deserved value as a sacred and powerful spiritual path.*

—TSULTRIM ALLIONE

was more fortunate than many because I knew that I wanted this child. For a man who feels ambivalence about assuming the responsibility of fatherhood or even about his commitment to the mother, it must be much more difficult. One point to keep in mind is that doubts are common and most men experience them.

Am I ready to be a father? Will this child interfere with my life? Can I afford this (another) child? Do I really want to be in a lifelong relationship with this woman? Will the child be healthy? It is okay to let yourself ask these questions and others. In fact, it is probably healthier in the long run to begin to face your shadows at the outset rather than to deny them. Many men report that becoming a father unleashed emotions and thoughts that were not usually part of their waking consciousness. You might find yourself, for example, reflecting more deeply on your own childhood and specifically on your father's place in your early years. Remember that pregnancy is a process that lasts nine months and that you have time to grow. At the same time, don't get lost in your doubts; don't forget to enjoy the moment, for the glow can grow faint at times.

Pregnancy produces some of the most profound changes to a woman's body and psyche that I can imagine. These changes are often so gradual that at any one moment they are imperceptible. The result is that it is often easy to forget what is really going on. We get so caught up in the stresses of day-to-day living that we forget we are in the midst of this extraordinary experience that is like nothing we have ever faced before. There are no simple road maps; no one person, not even this book, can fully prepare you for what lies ahead. If you expect the familiar, particularly if you are a first-time father, forget it.

## SUPPORTING YOUR PREGNANT PARTNER

Pregnancy requires surrender. Unfortunately, this word has negative connotations for most men in our culture. Surrender implies giving up to a stronger person or position; it implies defeat. This is decidedly not what I am trying to convey here.

To say that pregnancy requires surrender is to acknowledge and even honor the fact that the childbearing woman must—by biological necessity—accept that many aspects of her life are no longer under her control. It is a 24/7 task: twenty-four hours a day and seven days a week she is growing this baby inside of her womb. Everything about her life may be in a state of flux, of change. The predictable is fleeting, whether we are speaking of sleeping patterns, eating habits, emotions, or clothing styles and sizes. Anyone who has experienced pregnancy with his partner remembers the restaurant where she ordered a delectable meal, only to turn it away after the first bite. Or the new urgency in finding access to a public bathroom and in packing snacks for excursions out of the home, particularly in late pregnancy. In my many years of marriage to a practicing midwife, I have noticed that the women who do not surrender to these pregnancy changes, these new needs and desires, frequently have the most difficult transitions into birth and motherhood.

What does this mean for the new father? A number of years ago, I came across a slim volume entitled *Your Baby Is Your First Guru*. Translated literally, *guru* means "spiritual guide." The kernel of wisdom I gathered from this book is that learning to cheerfully accept the needs of your mate and baby, and to make them a priority in your life, develops your inner strength and your ability to face the ups and downs of life generally. We all know that life is not a straight line; we do not start and end, having traveled along a predictable path as in a board game. There will be crossroads of decision and detours as well as peaks and valleys. We will never have total control over all of the challenges life presents to us. We do have some measure of control over the attitude with which we face them. What better place to start than with our own mate and child?

At the same time, to surrender does not mean that fathers have to mimic the pregnancy experience itself. Although many men report sympathetic changes in their own biology during pregnancy—such as morning sickness, insomnia, and weight gain—the ideal model of partnership during pregnancy focuses on supporting the childbearing mother. Rather than mimicking her symptoms, we would be wiser to envision ourselves as the willow tree. Willows are renowned for their flexibility when the winds are gusting, yet they are rarely uprooted. Our task is to bend to our mate's needs, yet not to lose our sense of rootedness. Our mates will be looking to us throughout pregnancy, as well as during birth, for steadiness and reassurance. How can we provide these to her if we are so caught up in our own changes?

The downside is the danger that you may begin to feel unsupported. If mother and baby become the center of your universe, who will fill your needs? In the process, aren't you becoming henpecked, tied to your wife's apron strings, less of a man? Please know that the surfacing of resentments is a very common experience for expectant fathers. It would be surprising otherwise in a culture where male programming calls for men to be in control and to wear the pants in the family. Even those of you who are not bound by these stereotypes may feel resentful at times of the incredible amount of effort that pregnancy demands of your mate and thus of you.

Being pregnant together, in the fullest sense of the word *together*, does not mean that you and your mate have to do everything alike and at exactly the same time. As you nurture your partner, do not forget to nurture yourself. While pregnancy is not a time to go out to sow your oats in a last-chance fling at freedom, it is okay to continue to cultivate your interests and to meet your needs.

The key is to align yourself with your mate and baby in total love and understanding. Assume your full responsibilities as their protector. I know this notion may strike many as sex-role stereotyping, but my experience is otherwise. Becoming a father activates our protective instincts; most women want us to be protective at this time if for no other reason than they are incredibly preoccupied by the internal demands of pregnancy, including being fiercely protective of the child growing within them. But being protective does not mean that we have to dwell in the land of fight or flight. Perhaps *advocate* imparts a truer sense of our role than *protector*.

As an advocate, you are acting in the service of your pregnant mate to ensure that her best interests are always the priority. This requires your willingness to listen and to respond to her expressed needs. Even though male programming may tell you that you know better, you must maintain an open mind, affirm your mate's best intentions, and be fully prepared to yield to her requests. And, if necessary, you must offer your mate a gentle reminder when pregnancy calls on her to grow or change in ways she may resist or does not see. The fruits of this attentiveness and caring are a healthier mother and pregnancy, as well as improved communication and a deeper trust that will continue to nurture your relationship through the demands of raising a family together.

## BECOMING A PART OF THE PREGNANCY

Serving as an advocate allows fathers to assume an active and full involvement in the pregnancy process. This course of action requires the total involvement of both heart and mind. To act as an advocate, however, we must be knowledgeable about what we advocate. In other words, we must educate ourselves about pregnancy. Be truthful with yourself: how many of you have read this book carefully? I know that I knew very little about pregnancy and childbirth before the birth of our first child, despite having attended two home births previously and being married to a midwife. My life was busy; pregnancy was her field. Yet there is no way that I could advocate on behalf of Aviva and our babies if I didn't educate myself about the needs of pregnant women and the prenatal experiences of babies. When your partner puts those books in front of you, don't say "later." Turn off the television; quiet the music; put down your book. With all of the excellent material available today, which our forefathers didn't have access to, we have no excuse. If we remain uninformed, we are choosing to remain ignorant; what we are conveying is disinterest.

As you attune your mind to pregnancy, you can act from the heart with mindfulness. During pregnancy, loving your mate is the best way of loving your baby. In this dance, actions clearly speak louder than words, and it is often the simple, everyday actions that speak the loudest. Support your mate in caring for herself and the baby, for example, by bringing her a glass of fresh juice or water before she asks for it. Keep an eye on the refrigerator and ensure that it is well stocked with a variety of healthful foods. Exercise is something you can do together, whether it's a brisk walk or a session of yoga. Remember that pregnancy requires extra sleep. If your mate is at home full time, she might need to be reminded that it is okay to let the housework wait—she's not being lazy. Be resourceful: there are countless ways that you can show her that you recognize and appreciate all of her hard work growing your baby.

For those of you who already have children, the challenges can be far greater. I never realized how much easier the first pregnancy was until we experienced subsequent ones. With our first child, Aviva could eat and rest when her body signaled; in later pregnancies, she had to juggle the competing demands of children and the in utero baby. Fathers often have to be even more energetic in supporting these pregnant moms. There were times when I felt that coming home from work was like going to a second job. Fathers really need to be proactive with later pregnancies. Taking care of the children while your mate rests, preparing evening meals, pitching in with the housework—each of these acts serves not only to give her a break but to remind her that you care.

Be involved with your mate's prenatal care. This means more than just attending the regularly scheduled prenatal visits. Educate yourself about the various complications of pregnancy, and be ready to question a health care provider about any tests that are recommended. Pregnancy can activate many fears for a woman, especially about the well-being of her baby, and a father has a responsibility to deflect unwarranted pressures on his mate to submit to any procedures. The best health care providers welcome questions from fathers who are sincerely trying to become part of the pregnancy.

It is critically important that you continue to nurture your relationship with your mate. While this sounds easy, often you may get so busy with added responsibilities around the house that you forget to connect directly with her. You may even begin to feel imposed upon if, despite your contributions, she still wants to spend more time with you. Intimacy shared during pregnancy creates a reservoir of trust that can be drawn upon when you need it most—for example, during birth or after.

Massage is probably one of the easiest and most effective ways to connect two people, and its value in a healthy pregnancy cannot be overstated. You do not have to be a massage therapist to give a massage. More than anything else, what is required is sensitivity to your partner. Ask her what feels good, work lightly, and let her signal if she wants you to work harder on an area; give her the choice of using a massage oil or not. If you keep the lines of communication open and allow your heart to guide your hands, you will not go wrong. There is nothing that a pregnant mom enjoys more than to feel you loving your baby as you rub her belly. Gently stroke your child, even speak with him or her. What the child feels or hears perinatally is a question of current scientific research. My sense in the matter is clear: with each child, I felt a certain familiarity and bonding from the first moments after the birth. If nothing else, rubbing Aviva's belly on a regular basis gave me the confidence that our child felt truly loved and wanted by both of us and that I knew how to hold and touch him or her in nurturing ways.

By no means is this section exhaustive of the ways fathers can become a part of pregnancy. Needs and life circumstances vary. Through each of our four children, I feel that I have grown to be a more supportive and loving partner in pregnancy. But I have made mistakes, stemming primarily from an inability to listen and to yield to Aviva. I share this observation with you as both an encouragement and a reminder. It is possible to grow into the kind of man you envision and value, despite the lack of role models in our culture. In the process, you may inspire others and thereby contribute to the evolution of new models of manhood. Just remember that your opportunities to experience pregnancy are limited: most of us have only a handful of chances to be this close to the miracle of life. Cherish the occasion.

# PART II

# Common Concerns During Pregnancy

# CHAPTER 14

# A Guide to Common Pregnancy Issues

⋙⋘

*Pregnancy is a natural physiological process that,* if we are healthy, our bodies are quite capable of accomplishing. It is also a process that transforms our bodies and our lives, sometimes causing us discomfort! Your growing uterus will eventually cause your stomach to be displaced upward. This change, along with decreased gastric motility, can lead to heartburn. Women who work on their feet all day or who don't attend to keeping good posture or who have weak abdominal muscles may get severe backaches.

Many such discomforts common to pregnancy can be prevented, alleviated, or at least minimized. Also by nipping some symptoms in the bud—for example, constipation—we can prevent additional problems, for example, resultant hemorrhoids.

As a midwife and herbalist, I emphasize natural healing techniques. These are what I have experience using, and I've made every effort to present remedies that have been widely used with efficacy and safety. No deleterious effects are known to occur when the techniques described in this chapter are used as directed. When there may be a risk associated with a health concern, I have noted it and indicated the standard medical protocol currently in use. The descriptions of natural healing techniques in this chapter are also accompanied by any potential side effects. Always remember that any therapy—natural or otherwise—should be used carefully. Of course, every woman is unique, so please always give utmost attention to how you feel when trying anything new, and do consult your health care practitioner if you suspect a problem or need help in determining which treatment you should try. Refer to chapter 6 for more information on the safety of herbs during pregnancy.

May these suggestions assist you in enjoying a healthy and comfortable pregnancy.

# Anemia

Three types of nutritional anemias are most likely to occur during pregnancy: folic acid deficiency, known as *megaloblastic anemia*; pernicious anemia, which is a deficiency of vitamin B12; and iron deficiency anemia. In most cases, a healthy diet with appropriate supplementation will prevent and rectify nutritional deficiencies. Left untreated, anemia can lead to a variety of discomforts and medical problems for both mother and baby.

Your health care provider can help you to distinguish which you have and what various treatments might be appropriate for you.

## FOLIC ACID ANEMIA

Folic acid is one of the B vitamins. It is found primarily in leafy green vegetables as well as in wheat germ, molasses, nutritional yeast, whole grains, root vegetables, beans, milk, and liver. While theoretically we should be able to meet our folic acid needs from eating ample amounts of leafy greens and these other sources, about 30 percent of people possess a genetic alternation that interferes with optimal folic acid metabolism, and 10 percent have two alterations that lead to even further impairments in its metabolism. Folic acid is essential for healthy fetal neural development and may even play a role in the prevention of autism. All pregnant women should get 400 micrograms of folic acid or folate daily; women with either one or two of these *genetic polymorphisms* might need anywhere from 1 to 4 grams of *active folate (methylfolate)* daily. Discuss this with your midwife or physician. Adequate folate metabolism also plays a key role in the prevention of miscarriage and preeclampsia.

To obtain the maximum amount of folic acid from vegetables, eat them raw, steamed, or lightly sautéed. When vegetables are boiled, folic acid is leached out in the cooking water and most of it is discarded. Pregnant women should be certain to eat at least two large portions of leafy green vegetables daily as well as an ample amount of other foods that contain folic acid.

Symptoms of folic acid deficiency include a "mask of pregnancy" and other skin pigment changes, appetite loss, vomiting, persistent vaginal infections, and, because other B-complex vitamins may also be deficient, a host of nervous system complaints. Babies are more likely to be born with neural tube defects (such as spina bifida) when mothers are deficient in folic acid.

Herbs that contain folate acid include amaranth, watercress, parsley, chicory, nettle, dandelion leaves, and lamb's quarter greens. Most of these can be eaten as vegetables or steeped to make tea, though parsley should only be used in limited quantities as a vegetable, not as a tea, during pregnancy. However, using these is not a substitute for supplementation in pregnancy.

> CAUTION: **Parsley should only be used in limited quantities as a vegetable, not as a tea, during pregnancy.**

## VITAMIN B₁₂ DEFICIENCY

This deficiency is not common because vitamin B$_{12}$ is manufactured by bacteria in our intestines. It is stored in the liver and becomes available as needed by our bodies. We need only minute amounts daily, and that is usually available in most diets. However, several factors can lead to inadequate intake or absorption of this nutrient:

- A vegetarian diet that contains no dairy products may cause problems. It may take up to five years to use up stores of B$_{12}$ in the liver, and that long for a deficiency to appear.

- Stored B$_{12}$ may not cross the placenta (or breast milk), and therefore the baby may be deficient.

- Stomach acids that aid in the breakdown, absorption, and stimulation of B$_{12}$ production may be insufficient due to inadequate stomach acid production or a history of using antacid medications, particularly proton pump inhibitors (PPIs) such as Prilosec.

- Vitamin B$_{12}$ content may be depleted in foods produced by poor agricultural practices in soils that lack the mineral cobalt, an essential component of vitamin B$_{12}$. Nutrient loss in soils affects the levels of B$_{12}$ in both animal and vegetable foods.

- Many of us lack healthy gut flora, and an overgrowth of certain types of unhealthy gut flora compete with our own needs for the B$_{12}$ that we produce. If you have a lot of gas, bloating, or burping, you may need to supplement your B$_{12}$. Talk with your midwife or physician about small intestinal bacterial overgrowth if you have chronic B$_{12}$ deficiency.

Symptoms of vitamin B$_{12}$ deficiency include weakness and gastrointestinal disturbances such as loss of appetite and diarrhea; a sore tongue; slight yellowing of the skin; nervous system disturbances including soreness, weakness, or coordination problems in the fingers, arms, legs, and feet; diminished reflex response and sensory perception; difficulty in walking and speaking (stammering); and nerve deterioration. If you have these symptoms, you should seek medical diagnosis. Treatment of an existing B12 deficiency includes an injection of vitamin B12 twice in one year. It is considered safe, has no side effects, and is very effective. Left untreated, B12 deficiency can result in permanent mental impairment and paralysis.

You can usually get enough vitamin B12 by eating a wide variety of high-quality foods (particularly organically grown foods where there tends to be attention to soil quality), including ample amounts of vegetables, fruits, nuts, seeds, whole grains, and the regular consumption of some dairy products, preferably yogurt and hard cheeses, on a daily basis. Small amounts of meat on an occasional basis can ensure that you are also getting a concentrated source of the nutrient. Fermented foods such as miso and tempeh may contain small amounts of B12 and may also improve the intestinal production of this vitamin, which grows much like yeast and penicillin. Nutritional yeast can serve as a B12 supplement. Pregnant women need more B12 than nonpregnant women (see chapter 5). Adequate amounts may serve to prevent infection as well as aid in nervous irritability, memory impairment, depression, and insomnia.

## IRON DEFICIENCY ANEMIA

Iron deficiency anemia leads to a reduction in the oxygen-carrying capacity of our red blood cells. As a result, we may experience fatigue, dizziness, shortness of breath, general weakness, paleness (of the skin, fingernail beds, and mucous membranes), loss of appetite, heart palpitations, and gastrointestinal disturbances including constipation and abdominal pain. Frequent colds or infections may also be a sign that you are anemic. The cause of iron deficiency anemia is in most cases a nutritional deficiency; however, women who had super heavy or frequent periods prior to becoming pregnant may enter pregnancy with anemia. Anemia can also be caused by other problems, for example, sickle-cell disease, Thalassemia trait, other nutrient deficiencies, or a chronic infection.

Iron deficiency is common in women because we lose blood every month through our menses, and we often don't take enough time and care to replenish ourselves. Women may begin their pregnancies deficient in iron. Iron is essential during pregnancy for the adequate transport of oxygen through the mother and to the baby. The baby will store enough iron in its liver during the last couple of months of gestation to last for up to six months after birth. This is nature's way of assuring that the baby has enough iron reserves because breast milk is low in iron. If the mother is anemic, the baby may have insufficient iron stores and may also become anemic. Iron-deficient mothers may also have more difficulty with bleeding during birth than those who are well nourished and are more prone to fatigue and repeated illness as well as more susceptible to infection.

A simple blood test, done by just having your finger pricked by your midwife or physician and an on-the-spot analysis, can reveal your hemoglobin or hematocrit (depending upon the test performed), indicating whether you are anemic. If you are iron deficient, you may experience symptoms including pallor of the skin, fingernail beds, and the lining of the eyelids; weakness; fatigue and irritability; nausea and appetite loss (particularly when prolonged past the first trimester); constipation; shortness of breath; heart palpitations; pica (cravings for nonfood items such as cornstarch, clay, dirt, and ice); and an uncomfortable, restless feeling in your legs at night. Hemoglobin is the oxygen-carrying portion of the red blood cell. As the amount of blood plasma increases in midpregnancy, the concentration of hemoglobin decreases, causing the hemoglobin count to drop slightly, though the actual amount of hemoglobin in the blood has not changed. This is a desirable effect referred to as *hemodilution*. If the hemoglobin is below 11 milligrams in midpregnancy, herbal and nutritional approaches can be used to improve the levels. A low hemoglobin count (below 12 milligrams) in early or late pregnancy is considered indicative of anemia.

During the second trimester, at about twenty weeks, a pregnant woman's blood volume should expand to about 50 percent more than it was before. Most midwives feel that a hemoglobin count of 12 is ideal at the end of pregnancy. In fact, a high hemoglobin (over 13.5 milligrams) might actually be a sign of a contracted blood volume, in which case you may need to increase your protein, fluid, and salt intake. If this is the case, discuss the situation with your midwife or other care provider.

*Bonnie had fatigue, skin pallor, and shortness of breath. A blood test confirmed mild anemia. She began to increase her dietary iron and added herbal iron supplementation to her diet. Within a month, her symptoms were relieved and her blood tests normal. Her overall quality of life also improved dramatically as she began to have more energy and feel better.* ✺

You don't need to reduce your diet to numbers and milligrams to avoid iron deficiency anemia. Eating a well-balanced diet based on whole foods provides an excellent nutritional foundation. To ensure that you are obtaining adequate supplies of iron, eat iron-rich foods on a daily basis and choose from the selection of herbs that provide the extra boost you need. You can also use the following suggestions for the prevention and treatment of iron deficiency anemia prior to conception, throughout pregnancy, and after birth, especially if you've had any significant bleeding. If you are already anemic, you can expect to see noticeable improvement after two to three weeks of diligent work to build your blood.

## DIETARY RECOMMENDATIONS

- Iron supplements are hard for the body to assimilate and should not take the place of nutrient-rich foods. Therefore, it is important to include daily portions of iron-rich foods in your diet. These include dark green leafy vegetables, sunflower and pumpkin seeds, organic unsulphured dried fruits (raisins, prunes, black Mission figs, apricots, and cherries), blackstrap molasses, beets, red beans, dark turkey meat, and eggs. Beef contains a very highly absorbable form of iron called *heme* iron. A stew prepared with vegetables, organic beef, and a tomato base, eaten three times per week, can help to rapidly improve iron levels. Also, many of the plants listed under "Herbal Recommendations" below can be used as vegetables.

- Seaweeds, most notably kelp (kombu) and dulse, are very rich sources of iron. They can be eaten as vegetables (refer to macrobiotic cookbooks, available at natural food stores, for recipes); in powdered or flaked form, they can be sprinkled on foods; or, if you can't tolerate the taste, they can be taken in capsules. Take 1 to 2 tablespoons of flakes or powder, or approximately 8 "00" capsules daily.

- Take your iron-rich foods and iron supplements with vitamin C (250 to 500 milligrams of C each time you take your iron supplements, but do not exceed 2,000 milligrams per day). Vitamin C assists in the absorption of iron. Of course, all nutrients work in concert, so be certain that your overall diet is well balanced, too.

- Dairy products inhibit iron absorption, so have iron-rich meals and dairy-rich meals at different times. Don't take your iron supplements with dairy products.

- Caffeine and phosphates in soda interfere with iron absorption (and inhibit appetite, preventing adequate nutritional intake), so decrease your consumption or omit soda from your diet.

- Cooking in cast-iron pots increases the iron content of foods, so use them whenever possible.

- Regular exercise increases the body's demand for oxygen. This causes a response in the body that allows iron to be absorbed more easily, as iron occurs in the red blood cells as part of the oxygen-carrying process.

- If you do choose to take an iron supplement, use a chelated iron. (*Chelated* means that the mineral is chemically bound to another substance that the body can more easily absorb than the mineral itself, thus acting as a vehicle for the absorption of the mineral.) Ferrous gluconate, ferrous fumerate, and ferrous lactate are considered the most easily absorbable forms of iron.

- Iron supplements may be most easily digested when taken with a meal, particularly with dinner if you are prone to nausea earlier in the day.

  CAUTION: Commercial and prescription iron supplements may do more harm than good, particularly if they are causing constipation or other digestive upsets. In fact, I have often recommended that pregnant women discontinue iron pills because assimilating them is too taxing on the body. Herbal and dietary approaches to increasing your blood levels of iron are usually more effective.

## HERBAL RECOMMENDATIONS

- An excellent iron tonic for pregnant women is the humble herb nettle. My own preference is for a very dark green and strong-tasting infusion, made by steeping a large handful of the dried herb in 1 quart of boiling water for a couple of hours. If you prefer a milder brew, steep 3 to 4 tablespoons of the herb per quart of boiling water for thirty minutes. Drink between 1 and 4 cups daily depending on your needs.

- Liquid chlorophyll, usually derived from alfalfa, is another herbal source of iron. Take 1 tablespoon daily (not more unless so directed on the product label) as a supplement.

- Floradix Iron + Herbs is a supplement made from iron and extracts of dried fruits and herbs. It is delicious, easy to take, and can be purchased at most natural food stores. Many women have good results when using it along with the dietary recommendations and perhaps another of the herbal recommendations included here. Take according to the directions on the bottle.

- Chinese herbal formulas, such as dong quai and peony formula, can be beneficial for women with a history of anemia. Seek the assistance of a person trained in Chinese diagnosis and herbal prescription.

## Anxiety

(See "Insomnia and Anxiety" in this chapter.)

## Backaches and Sciatica

Pregnant women get backaches for many reasons: the weight of the baby and uterine contents placing stress on the lower back muscles, constipation, poor posture, standing for long periods of time, urinary tract infections, and the stress of overwork. Sciatica, a severe back pain that radiates into the legs, can occur from the growing baby and womb placing pressure on the sciatic nerve (located in the space between the hip bone and sacrum). In many cases, backaches and sciatica can be alleviated with the sensible use of exercise, nutrition, and herbs.

Pregnancy adds to the workload of your kidneys, which must filter both your wastes and your baby's wastes as well as maintain your expanding blood volume. The enlargement of your uterus can add physical pressure on the urinary tract, leading to infection, which in turn can cause backache. Speak with your care provider if you are experiencing backache—you may have a urinary tract infection.

### GENERAL RECOMMENDATIONS

- Good posture can prevent sciatic nerve discomfort and backache. Many pregnant women have a tendency to sway their bellies forward to handle the weight of the baby. This posture, known as *lordosis*, allows the lower back to sway forward, straining and eventually weakening the muscles in the lower back, leading to discomfort as well as strain on the abdominal muscles. Likewise, many women will slouch their shoulders forward, which leads to neck, shoulder, and upper-back discomfort.

- To improve your posture, and therefore greatly improve how you feel (your digestion will improve, and you will find it easier to breathe and eat), stand up very straight and tall—but not stiffly. Tuck your tailbone under so that your pelvis does not tilt forward and your back doesn't sway. Wear flat, comfortable shoes, and sit up straight in chairs and when you drive. Over time, good posture will become second nature to you because you will have strengthened your muscles. (See chapter 7, Exercise and Posture.)

- Take a walk every day and do exercises like leg lifts and lunges. Exercise is a great way to reduce both emotional and muscular tension and can significantly improve back problems. Swimming is a wonderful way to become weightless for a short time and get low-impact exercise. Yoga is useful for many problems. Many yoga centers now offer classes for pregnant women, and books and videos on pregnancy and yoga are readily available.

- Passionate lovemaking is great for relieving pelvic congestion, and if you rock your hips, you will also reduce lower back discomforts.

- Eliminating constipation is a must, because constipation can lead directly to lower backaches and pelvic discomfort. (See "Constipation" in this chapter.)

- Be certain that you are getting enough minerals from your diet. Insufficient calcium and magnesium, for example, can lead to muscle aches and a lowered threshold of discomfort. See chapter 5 for information on nutrition.

- Elevate your legs periodically, preferably for twenty minutes a day, to improve circulation in your legs. You can put your feet up on a chair or lie down and put them up on two pillows.

## HERBAL RECOMMENDATIONS

- Many herbs can reduce aches and pains. My two favorite herbs to be taken internally for deep backache and sciatica are skullcap and St. John's wort. Together these herbs form a dynamic duo that can be taken as a tincture, 30 drops of each, two to three times daily over the course of a few weeks, and, if necessary, a similar dose during acute discomfort. These tinctures can be added to a cup of hot chamomile or lemon balm tea for added relaxation and pain-reduction qualities.

- Black haw or cramp bark tincture can be taken to relieve backache. Use 25 drops of either, up to every half hour for two hours for acute spasm, or up to four times a day preventatively.

- Apply a combination of arnica and St. John's wort oils externally to relieve tension, promote healing of muscles, and reduce nerve tenderness, preferably having someone massage them into the affected areas. Put a warm water bottle over the treated area, and take time to consciously visualize yourself becoming loose and free of tension. You can do this daily. St. John's wort is said to contain substances that are able to penetrate to the endings of nerve fibers and promote their healing.

- Take a hot bath to which you have added Epsom salts or any of a number of essential oils or herbal infusions. Some possibilities are wintergreen, lavender, or rosemary oil; chamomile, lavender, or lemon balm; or a combination of these.

See sidebar below for two recipes for external use that you can easily make at home with wonderful results.

**WARNING: The herbs in these oils burn mucous membranes, so keep them away from sensitive areas such as your eyes. Essential oils are highly toxic if ingested, so store bottles out of the reach of children.**

### Deep-Ache Ointment

Melt ½ cup of coconut oil with 2 tablespoons sweet almond oil. Let cool slightly and add 1 teaspoon each of lobelia tincture, St. John's wort tincture, and cramp bark tincture. Pour into a clean, wide-mouth jar; let cool, cap and label it, and then apply as needed. This is one of the most effective oils I've found for deep aches, sprains, sciatica, frozen and stiff joints, and even arthritis. Use liberally as needed.

### Muscle Ache Oil

To 1 cup of olive oil, add ½ teaspoon of each of the following: cinnamon oil, spearmint oil, rosemary oil, and lavender oil. Shake vigorously and apply as needed. These oils stimulate circulation in the area to which they are applied, relieving circulatory congestion, promoting warmth, and inducing gentle muscle relaxation.

# Bleeding and Cramping in Early Pregnancy

Little is more disheartening than vaginal bleeding during pregnancy. Yet many women experience some bleeding during the first trimester, ranging from mild to heavy spotting, and they do not miscarry. Bleeding can occur after sexual activity or merely from a vaginal examination. Other causes include implantation of the fertilized egg in the uterine wall, bleeding caused by fluctuating hormonal levels occurring when you would normally have your period (some women will experience this for the first month or so of pregnancy and, very rarely, throughout the entire pregnancy), polyps on the cervix (if necessary, a physician can remove them), and a condition known as a *friable cervix* in which the tissue of the cervix is easily split. (This can usually be improved with a high-quality diet.)

The amount of bleeding you are experiencing can help you determine the type of care you should seek. If you are spotting or bleeding mildly, especially if the blood is brown, you can call your health care provider and ask for her opinion. Frequently you will be told to wait and watch for further possible signs of miscarriage (discussed below).

> **WARNING: If you are hemorrhaging (bleeding heavily and steadily—for example, soaking a large menstrual pad in a half hour or less), if you have been bleeding for a prolonged period of time, or if the blood is bright red (meaning that it is fresh blood), seek the help of your midwife or physician, or go right to the hospital emergency room.**
>
> **CALL EMS (911), or contact your health care support person and ask for her recommendations. If you are alone, contact your partner, a family member, friend, or neighbor so you have help if an emergency arises.**

If you feel your uterus cramping, it does not mean you will miscarry. There are other causes of cramping, including stretching of the round ligaments (that support the uterus), gas, constipation, and insufficient intake of calcium and magnesium. Cramping occurs in many pregnancies and, even when accompanied by spotting, does not necessarily mean that miscarriage is occurring.

*Lisa had a history of miscarriages and very much wanted to have this baby. Nonetheless, she began spotting and having contractions ten weeks into her pregnancy. She began regular consumption of an infusion to prevent miscarriage and, by twenty-four hours later, the symptoms had abated. One week later, she again began to spot and have mild contractions. She resumed the infusion and confirmed that the baby was still alive by having the baby's heartbeat listened to by a midwife who had a Doppler, which can detect heartbeat this early in pregnancy. She continued the infusion for another week, had no further problems, and gave birth to a healthy baby a few days after her due date.* ❮❮❮

Another lesser-known cause of bleeding and cramping during pregnancy is a urinary tract infection (UTI). I have seen several pregnant women bleed profusely and have regular uterine contractions caused by a UTI. Your lower abdomen or low back may ache, your urine may burn, and you may experience flu-like symptoms or malaise (depression and lack of motivation). You can have your midwife or physician check your urine (or check it yourself with urinalysis sticks) for the presence of leukocytes (white blood cells) or nitrites (a by-product of bacterial breakdown). The appearance of these together is a positive sign for a UTI and is a noninvasive method for testing. See "Urinary Tract Infections," later in this chapter, for treatment suggestions.

Perhaps the most dangerous cause of cramping in early pregnancy, sometimes accompanied by vaginal bleeding, is an ectopic pregnancy, which will be discussed later in this chapter.

## GENERAL RECOMMENDATIONS

- Try to calmly assess the situation and seek help—immediately—if necessary.

- Avoid intercourse, heavy lifting, and strenuous activity for several days after bleeding has ceased.

- Light massage may help relieve muscular cramping and spasms.

- If you are troubled by gas and constipation, you should address these complaints.

- If you determine that cramping is due to round ligament pain, gentle stretching can be effective. Touching your toes, lying on your back with your legs pulled up to your chest, or alternating toe touches while sitting with your legs stretched in front of you can all be effective.

## DIETARY RECOMMENDATIONS

- Be certain that you are getting enough minerals in your diet, especially calcium and magnesium, which are essential for the healthy functioning of muscular tissue and for preventing spasms. A dietary supplement may be in order if you are experiencing chronic problems, but your first recourse should always be to improve your diet.

- Excessive intake of dairy, particularly milk, may actually interfere with optimal calcium absorption and therefore should be avoided. Likewise, chocolate and caffeinated products (soda, coffee) inhibit absorption of calcium.

- For a cervix that tends to bleed or be lacerated easily or for a weakness of the placental bed, add 1,000 milligrams of vitamin C with bioflavonoids to your daily diet. Vitamin C plays an integral role in the health and strength of the blood vessels. To improve dietary intake of vitamin C, eat dark green leafy vegetables, raw cabbage, cantaloupe, strawberries, grapefruits, and oranges. Many of the foods you already enjoy may be rich in vitamin C; refer to chapter 5 for an extensive list.

- Make sure that you are taking your daily prenatal vitamin, and that it includes Vitamin E (alpha-tocopherol).

- According to traditional Chinese medicine, excessive cramping and bleeding can be caused by overconsumption of foods and beverages that are cold because they cause constriction of blood vessels and poor blood circulation. Examples of cold foods are those coming directly from the refrigerator or freezer as well as those produced in climates that are hotter than the one in which you live. For example, bananas and citrus would be considered extremely cooling for one who lives in New York, even more so in autumn or winter. It is also important to eat foods and drink beverages at room temperature or slightly warmed. Avoid cold beverages and foods such as smoothies and ice cream if cramping has been a problem.

## HERBAL RECOMMENDATIONS

- Black haw, cramp bark, and wild yam are all excellent antispasmodics that may be used safely during the first trimester to reduce cramping. Take $1/4$ to 1 teaspoon of one of the tinctures, or preferably a combination of black haw or cramp bark with the wild yam, up to every thirty minutes in the lower dosage, or every two hours in the higher dosage, depending on the frequency and severity of the cramping.

# Bleeding in Late-Pregnancy

With the exception of spotting in early pregnancy and blood-tinged discharge preceding or during labor, if you begin to bleed, call your midwife or physician immediately. If bleeding is profuse, call 911 or head to the nearest emergency room!

Sometimes a woman may see some streaks of blood in her vaginal mucus (on toilet tissue or underwear) after intercourse. This is no cause for alarm. It occurs if the cervix was slightly jarred. Bleeding later in pregnancy may be related to a placental problem, such as a placenta previa, a condition in which the placenta partially or completely covers the cervix, or a placental abruption, in which the placenta separates, to varying degrees, from the uterine wall. These two situations require immediate medical attention. A blood loss that causes you to soak a large menstrual pad within thirty minutes is termed a hemorrhage. All bleeding that occurs during pregnancy should be traced to the cause. Calm your mind, assess the situation, and be certain you and the baby are not endangered.

> CAUTION: Heavy or steady bleeding during the first four months of pregnancy usually signals a threatened miscarriage. Call your health care provider. See "Miscarriage" later in this chapter.

Always remember that even in an emergency room you can find caring and supportive people and that you can maintain your sense of power and authority over your body. Always bring a support person to act as an advocate for you when you seek medical care.

# Breasts, Sore

As early as the first few weeks of pregnancy, you may notice that your breasts are tender, sore, or tingly, and that your nipples are unusually sensitive. This is due to the usual breast enlargement that occurs as a result of hormonal changes accompanying pregnancy. It may remind you of those years in junior high school when your growing breasts were highly tender and sensitive. The hormones of pregnancy also help ready the breasts for breastfeeding. While the acute sensitivity usually subsides after a short time, your breasts, because of their increased size, may feel heavy and tender throughout pregnancy.

## GENERAL RECOMMENDATIONS

- When you are reclining, go braless to avoid constriction of your breasts and friction on your nipples.

- When you are out and about, particularly as you get farther along in your pregnancy, wear a bra that offers you support and helps prevent your breasts from feeling heavy.

- Hot soaks in the tub, with the water at a level over your breasts, can help to relieve discomfort and heaviness.

## HERBAL RECOMMENDATIONS

- For tenderness in early pregnancy, massage the following soothing and lovely scented oil into your breasts once or twice daily: To 3 ounces almond or melted coconut oil, add ½ ounce each of St. John's wort oil and arnica oil. Also add 5 drops each of lavender essential oil, rosemary essential oil, and rose geranium essential oil.

*Visualization is a wonderful tool for gently affecting physical change. Mary had been trying various techniques to change her baby to a head-down position, but to no avail. Her baby was consistently in a position where the shoulder was presenting. We decided to try a visualization—beginning with deep muscular relaxation. I then guided her through imagining her baby's head in her pelvis. We also told the baby that this head-down position would allow it to be born safely. By the end of the visualization, the baby's head had moved downward, and it stayed that way until her baby was born, vaginally and at home.*

# Breech Births

Breech births are not uncommon, but it is increasingly uncommon to find an obstetrician who knows how to deliver one vaginally. Because of this and some increased safety risks, most obstetricians only deliver breech babies—particularly with first-time moms—by cesarean. If you want to have your baby vaginally, and she or he insists on remaining breech, it's essential that you find a midwife or physician who is willing and skilled in performing vaginal breech births.

While most babies will have assumed their birth position by about thirty-six weeks, even some as early as thirty-four weeks, many babies will remain persistently breech only to turn a couple of weeks or even less, before the birth.

Rarely, a breech position occurs because of a congenital anomaly that prevents the baby from fitting head down in the pelvis, by a deformity or variation of the pelvis or uterus that prevents a head-down position, or by a short umbilical cord or one that is wrapped tightly around the neck. One of a set of twins is also often in a breech position. An ultrasound can usually clear up the reason for a breech presentation, if there is one, and can provide reassurance if you are planning a vaginal breech birth.

Because there is some small increased risk of problems for the baby with a vaginal breech birth, and because it can be difficult to find a birth provider willing to attend a vaginal breech, it is ideal to attempt to turn the baby prenatally. Here are some simple suggestions that you can try at home.

## SUGGESTIONS FOR TURNING A BREECH BABY

At thirty-two to thirty-four weeks, you can begin taking gentle measures to encourage your baby to turn head down:

- Moxibustion, a traditional Chinese treatment, is highly regarded and has recently been written up in the *Journal of the American Medical Association* for its ability to cause a breech baby to turn. It involves holding a lighted "cigar" made of the herb mugwort over a specific acupuncture point on the pinkie toe. This is done for ten to twenty minutes on each toe at a session. The heat stimulates energy in the point. The Chinese doctor from whom I learned this technique witnessed its effectiveness when his sister's baby was breech. I've since employed it and have found it useful as part of an overall approach but have done no studies on its effectiveness as a solitary treatment. It is simple to do and can be done at home.

  - You will need to purchase a couple of moxa sticks. Unless you purchase the "little-smoke" moxa sticks, perform the entire treatment in a well-ventilated room. Unwrap and remove the outer paper, leaving the inner white paper in place. Next, light the end of the stick with a match or candle and blow on the lit end until it glows like a coal. Hold the lit end one-half to two inches away from the outside edge of the little toe, near the toenail. It does not matter whether you begin on the left or right foot. Maintain the heat on the point for ten to twenty minutes; then do the same spot on the other foot. If at any time you feel a burning sensation, simply pull the moxa a bit farther away from the spot. Repeat this procedure twice each day until the baby turns.

- Spend time each day imagining your baby head down. Put pictures around your home of head-down babies in their mothers' bellies. Tell the baby that it's safe to turn and that it would help you relax if he or she would do so. Look closely at your own fears of birth and motherhood as well as any stresses in your life that might cause tight pelvic or abdominal muscles.

- Try pelvic tilts. Rest a board (any sturdy board of sufficient width to support you) at a 45-degree angle, putting one end on the floor and the other on the edge of a chair or sofa. Lie on the board with your head near the floor and your feet near the top of the board. Ten minutes in this position twice a day is the recommended length of time.

  CAUTION: Of course, you should not attempt headstands unless you are already adept at them.

- External version, in which hands on the mother's abdomen physically move the baby, is frequently an effective method, but it is not without risks and should therefore only be done by a skilled midwife or physician who can carefully monitor the baby's heartbeat while he or she is being turned. An ultrasound will be done before and during the procedure to be sure the baby does not become tangled in the umbilical cord in the turning process. If he or she is already wrapped in the cord, the procedure will not be attempted to avoid harming the baby. The procedure is not without significant risk and is therefore done in the hospital should an emergency cesarean be required.

Remember, if the baby does not turn despite all your efforts, and if neither you nor the baby seem to have a physical problem causing the breech or inhibiting birth, in all likelihood you will be able to birth your baby vaginally. Finding a supportive obstetrician or midwife will likely be the most difficult part of your job!

# Colds, Flu, and Mild Illnesses

Colds and flu generally pose no threat to the mom or baby as long as the mother remains well nourished with foods and fluids. During a severe illness—for example, with high fever (over 103°F), prolonged fever (longer than two or three days), or symptoms such as frequent and violent vomiting, diarrhea, and persistent coughing—it is wise to consult an experienced midwife or a physician. Herbs that you have used for treating colds when you were not pregnant may not be safe now, so refer to "Herbs to Avoid During Pregnancy" in chapter 6 before you begin any treatment.

Many women find that they have an increased resistance to illness and infection during pregnancy. Getting adequate rest, eating highly nutritious and natural foods, getting moderate exercise, and maintaining a generally adventuresome, positive outlook on life may go a long way toward keeping our resistance to illness strong. Yet this may be easier said than done if you are already busy with children, a career, or the many stresses that plague human beings in our fast-paced society. Anxieties about money, relationships, and time constraints can open the door to illness. Treatment of colds and other simple illnesses (such as an intestinal virus, for example) must therefore always include reflection on what is going on in your life that may have left you susceptible and what this illness can show you about your lifestyle that might serve you in the long run. This is not an invitation to blame yourself or anyone else; rather, it is an opportunity to be introspective and aware of your needs. Perhaps you can find practical ways to reduce stress in your life and create the space to care for yourself, your health, and your growing baby.

## GENERAL AND DIETARY RECOMMENDATIONS

- As soon as you feel the first signs of illness—fatigue, chills, loose bowels, or constipation—try to excuse yourself from your daily responsibilities and get some rest. This is the perfect time to turn off your telephone, ask for help with your kids, take a sick day (what I refer to as a "health day"—a day off to prevent yourself from getting really sick), and nurture yourself. Do what is comforting: take a warm bath with a few drops of relaxing oils such as lavender or rose and a few drops of antiseptic oils such as rosemary, thyme, or eucalyptus. The latter help clear respiratory congestion. Then put yourself to bed with a cup of hot herbal tea and perhaps a book you've been wanting to read (if it is relaxing), soothing music, or just a soft pillow and a cozy blanket and let yourself sleep. Fatigue is a prime reason for illness to occur, so let yourself rest as long as you feel you need to without feeling guilty.

- Often when we are ill, we lose our appetite. Indeed, this is the body's way of resting the digestive system and sending healing energy to other areas in your body. However, you still need to grow your baby. So if you don't feel much like eating, try broths, soups, and simple buttered toast.

A well-made vegetable soup, miso soup, or chicken soup can be as medicinal as any herbal remedy and is worth preparing. Add some rice or pasta and you will have nourishing, yet light food to sustain you until your appetite returns in a day or so.

- You must drink fluids, even if you must force yourself to do so. Your baby needs amniotic fluid, and your kidneys will be taxed if you don't drink adequately. In fact, you can even begin to have contractions if you get dehydrated. A full glass of clear fluid, broth, or tea every two hours if you are not feverish, and more if you are, is adequate. Keeping yourself well hydrated is essential when you are pregnant and is moreover an important component of healing from illness.

- Be certain to dress appropriately for the weather. If you are chilled, dress warmly, but don't become overheated. Wear breathable cotton clothing and cover yourself with natural-fiber blankets if at all possible. If your fever breaks in a heavy sweat and your clothes are wet and clammy, change them swiftly so you don't get chilled.

- Take about 250 milligrams of vitamin C every two hours, but don't exceed 2,000 milligrams daily during the first trimester; after that, don't exceed 4,000 milligrams daily. And discontinue either dosage of vitamin C after five days.

## HERBAL RECOMMENDATIONS

- Echinacea root tincture is a gentle but effective remedy for either a viral or bacterial infection. Combined with vitamin C, it is probably one of the best cold and flu preventions and treatments. It encourages the body's immune system to resist illness. Begin taking it at the earliest sign of sickness. Dosage is 1 drop of tincture for every 4 pounds of body weight (i.e., if you weigh 120 pounds you would take about 30 drops of tincture) every four hours for general prevention and mild colds. For more acute symptoms, you can either take the tincture every two hours or you can increase the dosage to 1 drop per 2 pounds of body weight. As you recover, slowly reduce the amount and frequency of the dosage. Echinacea has been demonstrated to be safe even for long-term use during pregnancy.

- Garlic lemonade is one of my family's favorite cold and flu remedies. An excellent bactericide, garlic is effective in treating all manner of general illnesses including colds, intestinal and stomach viruses, and strep throat. It can be taken in conjunction with echinacea and vitamin C.

- Ginger tea, also an excellent cold remedy, produces a warm feeling, preventing your temperature from getting too high and reducing tension. Ginger has properties similar to those of garlic. When made into a mild tea sweetened with lemon and honey, it has a very pleasant taste.

  **CAUTION: Ginger in large amounts (more than 1 to 2 grams a day) has been associated with miscarriage. Therefore, do not prepare it any stronger than directed and avoid it during the first trimester if you have a history of miscarriage.**

- Kudzu, an intruder into the southeastern landscape particularly here in Georgia where I live, yields a root high in starch, similar to arrowroot but more nutritious. This starch, available in small chunks and powder, makes an excellent tea that reduces fever, relaxes the muscles, eases stomach discomfort, and soothes inflamed mucous membranes in the throat and bronchial passages. Because of its high starch content, it is also nutritive. You can prepare kudzu root as a tea in a number of ways. I'll give you a couple of ideas, and you can choose what sounds appealing, even creating your own recipes as you go along. If you have an illness accompanied by diarrhea, you must be certain to drink enough fluid. Rehydration Drink (see page 200) is good for this.

- In addition to remedies already mentioned, you can drink a strong infusion of raspberry leaf tea during the second and third trimester of pregnancy made with 1 ounce of the dried leaves to 1 quart of water (steep for twenty minutes), taking $1/2$ cup every thirty minutes to one hour depending on the severity of the diarrhea. Raspberry leaves are notably astringent, tonifying the intestinal lining and reducing bowel discharge.

### Garlic Lemonade ✤

Steep 4 to 6 cloves of chopped raw garlic in 1 quart boiling water (cover the jar while you steep) for thirty minutes. Then add the juice of 1 or 2 lemons and honey or maple syrup to taste. Drink warm, up to 1 cup every two hours. If you don't find this tea palatable, try steeping the garlic as above, but add a couple of bouillon cubes or 1 tablespoon of miso to the tea instead of lemon and honey. This is a warming tea if you have chills but can be used at any time of the year.

### Ginger Tea ✤

Steep 1 teaspoon of freshly grated raw ginger in 1 cup boiling water for fifteen minutes. Steep covered to retain the volatile oils, which are antiseptic. Sweeten and add lemon if desired. You can take a hot cup of this tea every two hours. It is also soothing for a sore throat and eases respiratory congestion.

### Garlic-Onion-Ginger-Kudzu Tea ✤

This is really more of a soup, taught to me by an acupuncturist friend, and is one of my personal favorites when I feel a cold coming on or if I feel chilled. Sauté $1/2$ onion, 2 cloves of chopped fresh garlic, and $1/2$ inch of chopped fresh ginger root in 1 tablespoon of olive or sesame oil for two to three minutes. Add 3 cups of water, cover, bring to a boil, and simmer for about twenty minutes. Then add 1 tablespoon of miso paste and stir. In a small cup, dilute 2 teaspoons of kudzu starch in $1/4$ cup cold water (if you try to do this in hot water, it will form gelatinous clumps that will not dissolve). Add the starch to the broth, stirring constantly for two minutes. Turn off the heat and drink when it is warm but not hot. Use this freely throughout the day, preparing more as needed.

# Constipation

This is a very common problem for pregnant women because (1) it is widespread in our society; (2) pregnancy hormones decrease bowel activity and tone; (3) the growing baby and womb place pressure on the intestines and rectum, sometimes making bowel movements more difficult; (4) iron deficiency, common during pregnancy, leads to constipation; and (5) commercial iron supplements can cause constipation because they are so hard to assimilate.

Constipation is avoidable and, with direct attention, easily remedied.

## GENERAL RECOMMENDATIONS

- Get more exercise. A brisk walk each day, especially at the same time, can be a great boost to your digestion and promote regular evacuation. Many yoga exercises are also beneficial.

- Give yourself time each day to sit on the toilet. Relax and wait patiently, breathing deeply and possibly tightening and relaxing your anal muscle a few times to stimulate a bowel movement. The body has regular intervals for elimination, and if you don't go when you get the urge, the urge will pass and the stool will be retained. The longer it sits in there, the harder it will be to eliminate later on. Avoid straining as it will lead to hemorrhoids.

- Squatting is the physiologically natural position for bowel movements; therefore, getting up and squatting on the seat (no kidding!) can facilitate the process. If you can't handle this idea, at least put your feet up on a low stool or on the side of the bathtub while you try to go.

- Recline on your bed or, if possible, in a warm bath. Massage your abdomen deeply in a clockwise direction, starting at the "six o'clock" point and circling back around to it. Do this for ten or fifteen minutes before you return to the toilet.

## DIETARY RECOMMENDATIONS

- Eat an abundance of high fiber fresh vegetables, particularly various lettuces, kale, and collard greens. Eat raw vegetables with meals and snacks. You should have at least two large portions of raw vegetables each day.

- Cut back on cheese, meat, and highly fatty foods.

- Drink adequate amounts of water. Warm water with lemon first thing in the morning can be helpful.

- Magnesium citrate, at a dose ranging from 300 to 800 milligrams daily, can relieve constipation. Start at the lower dose and increase to the maximum dose as needed to achieve a well-formed daily stool.

- Yogurt (live culture), if you tolerate dairy, or a probiotic can also help eliminate constipation and populate the intestines with flora necessary for healthy bowel functioning.

## HERBAL RECOMMENDATIONS

- The most effective and safest remedy for use by pregnant women is a syrup of dandelion and yellow dock roots in a base of blackstrap molasses. Ironically, this same preparation is used for treating iron deficiency anemia. Unlike typical iron supplements, which are constipating, this natural remedy is iron-rich and also treats constipation—itself a sign of anemia. These herbs help move the energy of the bowels gently downward without stimulating the uterus.

- Senna tea can be taken occasionally for constipation but is best not taken daily. Combine 1 teaspoon of senna leaves and 1/2 teaspoon of spearmint. Steep in 1 cup of boiling water for ten minutes. Strain and drink 1 to 2 cups. A bowel movement will usually ensue about eight hours later, so taking this before bed can be great timing to ensure a first morning bowel movement.

  **CAUTION: Herbal laxatives including buckthorn, aloes, and castor oil can cause labor to begin as they stimulate the bowels.**

  **WARNING: Some may also be harmful to the baby's development, affecting the central nervous system. Therefore, avoid the use of all purgatives during pregnancy.**

*At the time of her first visit, Molly was anemic, irritable, tired, and severely constipated, made worse by the double dose of iron supplements her OB gave her. She hadn't had a bowel movement in two weeks when we first met, and you can imagine, at 32 weeks pregnant, this didn't make her feel too comfortable. She began to increase her fruit and vegetable intake, added oat bran to her daily diet, stopped the iron supplements, and instead started taking Floradix iron and herbs. Within a short time she was having a daily bowel movement, making her a much happier camper. And with the more natural iron supplementation, her anemia resolved, and along with it her irritability and fatigue.*

### Morning Chia-Lax
To make a morning laxative, soak four dried, pitted prunes and 2 teaspoons of chia seeds in 1/2 cup of warm unfiltered apple juice for ten minutes. Eat and drink all of the prunes, chia seeds, and juice.

# Cramping

(See "Bleeding and Cramping in Early Pregnancy" in this chapter.)

# Depression

(See "Emotional Swings" in this chapter.)

# Ectopic Pregnancy

Ectopic pregnancy means a pregnancy where the baby does not lie within the uterine cavity. Most commonly it occurs in a fallopian tube but may also occur elsewhere, including in the abdomen or an ovary. Ectopic pregnancies are extremely dangerous, because when they rupture, they can lead to sudden, life-threatening hemorrhage and shock. Part of what makes them so dangerous is that the symptoms may be subtle until rupture occurs, and then the situation becomes an emergency. Before this, a woman may not even realize that she is pregnant, let alone that the pregnancy is ectopic.

Certain factors may increase the likelihood that an ectopic pregnancy will occur, including pelvic infections (especially pelvic inflammatory disease [PID]), abortions, endometriosis, prior pelvic surgery, use of an IUD (intrauterine device), previous ectopic pregnancies, or any condition that may have caused scarring or adhesions in the pelvic organs.

Possible symptoms alerting you to an ectopic pregnancy include an unusually early, late, missed, or spotty period; abdominal pain that can be dull or intensely sharp; and irregular vaginal bleeding. When there is a rupture, the pain usually becomes severe, gets progressively worse, and most often is located on only one side of the lower abdomen. Other signs may include pain on only one side that may radiate into the arm, shoulder, chest, or upper back; scanty brownish bleeding that is intermittent; and eventually signs of shock, which include dizziness, anxiety, shortness of breath, clamminess of the skin, fainting, and pallor.

> WARNING: Ectopic pregnancy is a life-threatening emergency requiring immediate medical care. Alternative therapies do not apply!

Usually surgery will be required, and ideally it can be done before the rupture occurs. Most physicians make every effort to repair the tube or ovary, but it may need to be removed; ask whether surgery is the only option.

It is important for you to explore and allow whatever feelings arise because this a frightening medical emergency and it may mean the loss of your baby. National and local support groups dedicated to helping families cope with pregnancy loss can be a great source of comfort and aid during this time.

## Edema

(See "Swelling" in this chapter.)

## Emotional Swings

Pregnancy is certainly a time of great change for women, both in its physical challenges and in the new responsibilities it brings. It is a time when our bodies are circulating high levels of hormones and demanding a very good diet. Combine all of these factors, and it is not surprising that pregnant women find themselves experiencing highs and lows with great rapidity, even in the course of minutes. Add fatigue, the possibility of an unwanted pregnancy, anxieties about the baby's health, the prospect of motherhood, worries about how to maintain a job and care for a baby, an increasing body weight and a changing body shape in a culture that values thinness, not to mention the general discomforts of pregnancy, and it is even less surprising that pregnant women feel bouts of depression and insecurity. I'm always amazed at how easily I cry over sappy sentimental songs when I'm pregnant, and at how joyful I feel when I see buds opening in the spring and other simple miracles of life.

Pregnancy seems to be a key that unlocks doors to old experiences and feelings, particularly those regarding relationships that have had great impact on us, most notably our relationships with our mothers. For some women, the availability of their mothers as a source of support and information is comforting and valuable, but for others, proximity to our mothers can be a source of pain and conflict. For all women, pregnancy causes us to reflect on how we were raised and how we may want to raise our children similarly or differently. Reflecting on childhood can be confusing or painful, but it also offers new opportunities for personal growth. Finding ways to heal painful feelings can be productive, enabling us to move into motherhood with a fresh perspective. Moreover, such reflection may allow you to enjoy extended family support.

How your partner reacts and responds to your pregnancy can influence how you feel about yourself, particularly if you are dependent on your mate for financial

*Audrey's third baby was still breech just a week and a half before it was due. During this time, she was experiencing a lot of personal stress—her husband's business wasn't going well, she was overwhelmed by her two children (both under four years old), and she had recently been told some birth horror stories by a neighbor. At a prenatal visit, she opened up and shared all of these worries and had a healthy cry. Within a day, her baby changed to a head-down position and was born after a labor of a few hours. Perhaps this was coincidental—or perhaps letting go of her tensions, which were affecting her pelvic and uterine muscles, provided more room for her baby to change position.* ✺

(or other) support. Even if you are not financially dependent, if your partner finds your changing body unattractive, for example, you are likely to feel very hurt. If your partner seems disinterested in feeling the baby move, or if he refuses to share in your joy, you may experience rejection, sadness, or a sense of being "in it" alone.

Pregnant women are culturally expected to, and thus "allowed to," have periodic emotional outbursts, be subject to strange whims and cravings, and be somewhat irrational, but we are also expected to be in a state of joyful anticipation about the coming baby—to have a certain pregnancy "glow." Our culture also characterizes  symptoms of emotional problems. As a result, a pregnant woman may feel obligated to keep these feelings to herself or dismiss them as "normal emotional outbursts." The problem is that we may be disregarding issues that need some attention. We should tell our mates that we feel rejected when they are disinterested in the baby, or when they do not find our growing bodies attractive. While we may still feel these heightened emotions after such a discussion, we probably will be better able to cope. In addition, when we assume that extreme emotional sensitivity is normal in pregnancy, we may overlook nutritional or other physical factors that can contribute to the unpleasantness of being on an emotional roller coaster.

## GENERAL RECOMMENDATIONS ✺

- I cannot overstate the importance of excellent nutrition from both food and herbal sources, as well as adequate rest and exercise. Read chapters 5 through 8 thoroughly for a full discussion of these topics.

- Stable blood sugar can help you maintain a stable mood. Avoid caffeine and sugary foods, which lead to sugar crashes; keep blood sugar stable with frequent meals and small snacks rich in high-quality protein and good-quality fats, every three to four hours. Don't skip meals or allow your blood sugar to dip.

- Stay well hydrated. Inadequate fluid intake can affect your mood, making you feel more irritable, tired, or depressed.

- Accepting, not dismissing, your feelings is important. This means that you recognize and acknowledge what is bothering you. If you feel worried about birth, you don't have to dwell on gruesome details of rare complications or imagine yourself in some horrible scene from a TV emergency room. You can say to yourself, "Okay, I am afraid about birth." Try to find a source for your fear; ask yourself where this anxiety arises from. Perhaps as a young child you knew someone who had problems or you've heard frightening birth stories. By recognizing the source of your fear, you can separate it from your own personal experience.

- If you are afraid of a particular complication, you can ask your midwife or physician how she deals with it. Becoming more educated will often decrease your anxiety. If your issues relate to other matters, such as relationship problems with your mate, body-image anxieties, or financial worries, try to find constructive ways to address and resolve them. Midwives often help women work through a wide variety of issues, so speaking with your midwife, if you have one, can be helpful and comforting. A close friend or a counselor can also be a good listener and help you get to the bottom of your fears.

- Be true to yourself and deal with your problems to the best of your ability. If you find yourself in a situation that makes you feel bad, it is fair either to change the situation or extricate yourself from it. For example, if other women start to tell you awful stories about birth, it is perfectly reasonable to excuse yourself from the discussion or make it clear that the discussion disturbs you and you don't wish it to continue. You can't always wait for people to read your mind—sometimes you must make your needs known and stand up for yourself.

- Keeping a journal is an excellent way to give voice to your emotions. It can also provide a time of quiet reflection on a regular basis. You can create a nice ritual for yourself: drink a cup of relaxing herbal tea in your favorite cup, listen to soothing music, and write your thoughts, feelings, and impressions. This can be a welcome release from which you emerge refreshed. The act of writing can help you work out and resolve concerns. There are several books available on journal writing, some written specifically for women; inquire at your local bookstore for titles.

- Allow yourself to be human, accepting all the ups and downs we must go through. Don't give yourself the double whammy by feeling bad about feeling bad. Guilt doesn't get you anywhere in this situation. Feel what you feel and move on—you don't have to psychoanalyze yourself or explain or justify your feelings. How you feel is simply how you feel.

- Try to appreciate your heightened sensitivity. Being attuned to subtle emotional nuances in your interactions with others and to your own emotions can give rise to a deep empathy that will help you understand the subtle messages and feelings that your baby will need you to interpret after birth. When babies' subtle cues are heeded, they frequently have less need to resort to crying to get their message across. Many times crying is a strong way of expressing something that wasn't picked up through more subtle communications. Daily time for reflection and journal writing enhances your consciousness.

- Creative forms of expression can provide a welcome outlet for your emotions. Painting, drawing, sculpting, dancing, or singing can transform inner tensions.

## DIETARY RECOMMENDATIONS

Depression and other difficult emotional states can result from nutritional deficiency as well as lack of exercise.

## HERBAL RECOMMENDATIONS

- Passionflower has marked benefits for pregnant women with extreme mood swings, particularly anxiety and irritability. Use as a tincture, 10 to 30 drops up to three times daily.

- The general comfort of a warm bath enhanced with a few drops of essential oil of rose or lavender, or a massage with diluted oils of rose, lavender, St. John's wort, and chamomile are very helpful. To promote a more restful sleep and to reduce irritability when you wake, try sleeping on an herbal pillow stuffed with chamomile or lavender blossoms, or sprinkle a few drops of these oils on your pillow or put them in a diffuser next to your bed.

### Calming Tea 🌾

Combine 1 teaspoon chamomile flowers, 1 teaspoon lemon balm, and $^1/_2$ teaspoon lavender flowers, steep in 1 cup boiling water (covered) for ten to fifteen minutes, strain, and drink warm, with honey if you prefer. Do this as often as you wish throughout pregnancy for stress, indigestion, sleeplessness, and anxiety. You can also take this tea during labor to help you ease discomfort from contractions. A worthwhile additive to your medicine pantry, it is simple to prepare and delicious.

### Stress-Free Formula 🌾

- 1 ounce passionflower tincture
- 1 ounce skullcap tincture
- 1 ounce fresh milky oats tincture
- $^1/_2$ ounce chamomile tincture
- $^1/_2$ ounce lavender tincture

Combine all the tinctures and take 20 drops of this mixture every fifteen to thirty minutes for up to two hours before bed to promote rest and relief from anxiety.

# Fatigue

It is completely normal to need more sleep during pregnancy. Your body is working overtime. As my close friend, also a midwife, says, "It's a time of heavy construction." By the end of your first trimester, you have helped your baby develop all of his or her body parts, and that is an incredible accomplishment! In addition to all this building work, your own body and psyche are undergoing great changes and adjustments.

## GENERAL RECOMMENDATIONS 🌾

- Getting more sleep now that you are pregnant is important. Your emotions will be steadier, your digestion easier, and you will be less susceptible to infections, constipation, headaches, and morning sickness. Lack of sleep can lead to depression, irritability, and weepiness.

- You may, in fact, find yourself taking naps or dozing off in a chair at eight o'clock in the evening. Learn to listen to your body and your need to rest. Try not to worry about all that you are "not getting done."

- Stress, a job outside of the home, or older children to look after can further increase your fatigue. Women who have had children close together and are still nursing a toddler or keeping up with the needs of a family are particularly prone to exhaustion. This fatigue can ebb and flow. To minimize this, permit yourself to rest when you can, and prioritize your activities. For example, if housekeeping can wait, rest when you might otherwise be cleaning.

- Exercise, especially in the fresh air, is an excellent way to increase your oxygen intake and improve your circulation, appetite, and bowel function. Your depression will lift, and insomnia and restless sleep will lessen. Even a brisk walk at least three times a week can make a tremendous difference in your well-being. A gentle toning exercise such as yoga can help wash away fatigue.

- Getting a massage can be relaxing and invigorating. If you can't afford a professional massage, have your mate or close friend give you one (or ask your midwife to massage you at prenatal sessions).

- When you need help, be sure to ask for it.

## DIETARY RECOMMENDATIONS

- If you find yourself persistently irritable and exhausted, this may be a symptom of a nutritional problem. Frequently, this type of deep exhaustion is accompanied by some of the following symptoms: general weakness, pallor, shortness of breath, nausea ranging from mild to severe, dizziness, heart palpitations, and lack of appetite. See "Anemia" (in this chapter) for natural therapies that can help you obtain enough iron in your daily diet. When there is insufficient iron in your diet, your body is not getting enough oxygen and you may feel fatigued.

- Be certain that you are eating regularly and getting enough protein and complex carbohydrates. These are nutrients that provide your body with a steady source of energy and keep your blood sugar balanced.

## HERBAL RECOMMENDATIONS ⫷

- Stimulants—even herbal ones—should not be used during pregnancy.

- Take a strong nettle infusion, 2 to 3 cups per day, to nourish the adrenals, regulate blood sugar, improve nutrient intake, and build iron levels. To prepare, steep 4 TBS dried nettle leaf in 1 quart of boiling water for 1 hour, strain and drink this lovely green infusion, 1 to 2 cups per day. The remainder will keep in the fridge for 24 hours.

- Use Iron Tonic Syrup (see below) to boost iron levels if fatigue is associated with anemia.

- Herbal baths can be invigorating, refreshing the mind and spirit and reducing fatigue and depression. Add 3 to 5 drops of an essential oil to your bath. Good choices are peppermint, lemon, orange, sandalwood, and rosemary oils. Splash mildly cool water on your body after the bath and settle in for a peaceful rest. Alternatively, if you don't have time for a full bath, add 2 to 3 drops of oil to a basin of cool water and splash yourself with the invigorating scents—a sure, quick energy-pickup!

  CAUTION: **Never use essential oils internally.**

### Iron Tonic Syrup Recipe ⫷

Commercial iron supplements are frequently hard to digest and can cause constipation. This iron tonic is easy to digest and is even a gentle, natural laxative. It also provides other trace minerals, strengthens the liver and digestive system, and enhances the body's overall assimilation of nutrients.

- $1/2$ ounce dried yellow dock
- $1/2$ ounce dandelion roots
- 1 pint boiling water

Combine the herbs in a glass jar. Add the water, cover, and steep the herbs for 4 to 8 hours. Strain the liquid into a small saucepan and reduce by simmering to 1 cup of liquid. Add $1/2$ cup of honey or a combination of honey and molasses (molasses increases the iron value). Let cool to room temperature and store in a bottle in the refrigerator. The tonic keeps up to 2 weeks in the fridge.

   To use: Iron tonic syrup is for children 2 years and older. The dosage is 1 to 3 teaspoons daily for children, 1 to 2 tablespoons daily for teenagers and adults.

# Gestational Diabetes

Gestational diabetes mellitus (GDM) is a condition that develops during pregnancy when the body is not able to make enough insulin or is resistant to the insulin that is being made. Women who develop gestational diabetes in pregnancy have a 50 percent chance of becoming diabetic later in life, and diabetes in pregnancy increases risks of heart malformations in the baby, can lead the baby to develop serious low blood sugar after birth, and increases the baby's risks of being born too large, necessitating a cesarean section. Additionally, babies born to diabetic mothers also have a higher risk of becoming diabetic later in life.

Prenatal glucose testing for pregnant women is not routinely done in many European countries, and, in the first edition of this book, I discouraged routine use of this test. However, diabetes in pregnancy truly does increase risks to mother and baby, and since the publication of the first edition of this book nearly two decades ago, rates of obesity have skyrocketed along with rates of diabetes.

So, although there is overwhelming evidence that the use of *routine* glucose testing for pregnant women is an unnecessarily invasive procedure that is best reserved for situations in which the need for the test is clearly indicated, there are some people for whom such testing is appropriate: women with a history of diabetes, a strong family history of diabetes, a history of polycystic ovarian syndrome, and women who are overweight at the start of or during pregnancy can be considered appropriate candidates.

A diet that keeps blood sugar well controlled is both the optimal prevention and treatment of gestational diabetes. While not studied for safety during pregnancy, cinnamon is an herb that is generally considered safe in pregnancy and which may help to control blood sugar—usually in a dose of 1 teaspoon per day which can be taken in capsules or in food. Other supplements commonly used to help with blood sugar control have not been tested for pregnancy safety. Therefore, working with a midwife or physician highly skilled in treating gestational diabetes with a natural approach, and with a nutritionist to create an optimal diet is the best way to address this problem. Because of the potential risks to the baby of untreated diabetes in pregnancy, if blood sugar cannot be controlled with diet, insulin is an appropriate consideration. After pregnancy, and even while breastfeeding, if elevated blood sugar persists, a wider range of herbs and supplements can be considered.

# Headaches

Headaches can stem from a number of causes, most commonly stress, tension, fatigue, dehydration, low blood sugar, constipation, dehydration, inadequate protein intake, or dietary insufficiency of minerals (particularly calcium and iron). Women prone to headaches before pregnancy may continue to have headaches during pregnancy, and women who are unable to nurture themselves adequately may develop headaches.

> **WARNING: Severe headaches beginning suddenly after the sixth month of pregnancy can signal preeclampsia, so check with your midwife or physician and care for yourself accordingly (see "Preeclampsia" in this chapter.). Untreated, preeclampsia can become a life-threatening condition. Severe headaches that increase in frequency and pain or that occur in women who are not prone to them can be a sign of a serious problem requiring immediate medical assistance.**

## GENERAL RECOMMENDATIONS

- Stress causes you to contract your muscles, reducing blood flow and making your body function less effectively.

- Sometimes fatigue can lead to tension headaches, so be sure that you are sleeping enough, and whenever possible, take a nap.

- Creative visualization is useful. Begin by choosing a comfortable spot in which you can sit or stretch out for as long as you are able, or for at least ten minutes. Get comfortable. Close your eyes and allow the tension to melt away, beginning at your feet and slowly working up your body until you reach your head. The different parts of your body should become progressively looser, as if you are floating on water. You can imagine hands massaging you deeply, lightly, or however you prefer. Imagine yourself basking in this relaxed state. Allow your mind to travel then to an environment that comforts, relaxes, and nourishes you. Choose a favorite image—walking on the beach, floating in a luxurious bath, or sinking deeply into a featherbed. When you feel calm and relaxed, open your eyes and slowly come back.

- As you relax, specifically focus on any images that may tell you the cause of the headache or possible remedies. When we enter deep states of relaxation, we are often able to access information that is not immediately available to us in our waking consciousness. You may see images of tension or experience fears about pregnancy or birth. By becoming aware of tension and its source, we can take steps to resolve it. Relaxation tapes for pregnant women are available, or make your own using the visualization suggestions in chapter 8.

- Constipation is a common cause of headaches. Substances that your body needs to eliminate are reabsorbed. At least one bowel movement daily can relieve headaches as well as prevent other health problems. See "Constipation" (in this chapter) for more information.

## DIETARY RECOMMENDATIONS

- Poor nutrition with resulting hypoglycemia can cause headaches. High-protein, high-carbohydrate snacks can help.

- Dehydration can also cause headaches, so drink enough fluids throughout the day, at least a tall glass of water or a nutritious beverage every few hours. You may feel parched, depressed, or hot if you aren't drinking enough. You may notice that you have some contractions, known to occur when pregnant women become dehydrated. You can reverse all these symptoms by eating and drinking adequately throughout the day.

- Caffeinated beverages (such as coffee and soda) and chocolate can cause headaches. Try to avoid them.

- Iron deficiency may lead you to have headaches, as will protein deficiency.

- You may need to add more calcium and magnesium to your diet. Refer to chapter 5 for dietary recommendations and consider adding a supplement containing 600 to 800 milligrams of calcium and 300 to 400 milligrams of magnesium.

Many nervine herbs are effective for soothing tension headaches. Nervines are gentle herbs used to soothe and calm the nervous system. Herbs that can be used as teas include chamomile, lemon balm, catnip, and lavender. You can take these herbs singly or in a combination of two or three in tea form, taking several cups daily. For more severe headaches, use these as tinctures, and also add either or both cramp bark or passionflower. You can also use a combination tincture of equal parts of each of these herbs, with the addition of either cramp bark or passion flower tincture also in equal measure. The dose is 20 to 40 drops of the tincture (depending on severity of the headache) added to an herbal tea or ¼ cup of warm water. Repeat one to two times in fifteen minutes and, if needed, fifteen minutes later, to maximize effectiveness. If the headache is more severe than usual, accompanied by visual disturbances, elevated blood pressure, abdominal pain, or other unusual symptoms, or seems to be more than a tension headache, please contact your obstetrician or midwife immediately.

### Relaxation Tea 🌿

A formula that I enjoy for relaxation during pregnancy contains 1 teaspoon chamomile flowers, 1 teaspoon lemon balm, and ½ teaspoon lavender flowers. Steep this mixture in 1 cup of boiling water for ten minutes (covered) and drink hot.

# Herpes

This section discusses type 2, genital herpes, though the recommendations are also applicable to type 1, oral herpes.

Herpes is a viral infection that, once contracted, stays dormant in the nerves located at the base of the spine. This infection will flare up when triggered by stress, fatigue, and dietary deficiencies. A woman who becomes infected with herpes for the first time during pregnancy, and particularly when she is close to the time of birth, may miscarry, or the baby may develop congenital anomalies or become very sick. It is therefore essential that you know whether your sexual partner has ever been exposed to or had herpes.

Women who had herpes before becoming pregnant are at minimal risk for passing the infection on to the baby prenatally because they have developed antibodies to the virus that protect the baby. But there is a risk of passing a herpes infection on to the baby if a mother gives birth with active genital sores, and this can cause the baby to develop a serious and even life-threatening infection; for this reason, a cesarean section is a standard procedure for women in the United States with active herpes at the end of pregnancy. This is a matter of debate among obstetricians: European physicians claim that herpes is a fairly low risk for the baby compared to the higher risk of a cesarean section. But most American doctors are not yet convinced of the safety of vaginal birth with active herpes lesions. Obviously, this will be a decision that requires a good deal of thought and the support of your birth attendant. A home birth is not recommended if you have active herpes at the time of birth or in the week prior.

The symptoms of a herpes outbreak usually begin three to five days before the sores appear: flu-like feelings, aching in the genital area, tingling or itching where the sores will erupt, emotional irritability, and sometimes painful urination or swollen lymph nodes. The lesions begin as small blisters that turn into small sores that then crust over and heal. There can be one lesion or many, and they can appear on either the external or internal parts of the genitals, including the cervix. The infection is contagious during the entire range of symptoms, so sexual activity should be discontinued at the earliest sign of any symptom until the sores are completely healed and are no longer visible. This can take up to a couple of weeks.

Herpes is quite common. I've worked with a number of women with a history of herpes, including one woman who had two previous cesareans. She went on to have her third baby at home with no lesions present. Most people have a "body barometer," a physical symptom or syndrome that pops up at times of stress. It could be an old injury site that begins to ache, a headache that develops when you have a deadline, or herpes that flares up. These are messages that you are dealing with too much internal pressure. By learning to recognize the early signs of stress, we can learn to slow down. If you anticipate a stressful time coming, you can take measures that prevent an outbreak; and if you do notice prodromal (preherpes) symptoms, you can begin to use herbs, address the stress, and improve your diet. You can get to the point where you rarely, if ever, have another herpes outbreak.

## GENERAL AND DIETARY RECOMMENDATIONS

Sexual partners with herpes can also follow the recommendations here.

- Stress reduction will help prevent herpes outbreaks. Make sure you are resting enough, and address any sexual issues that may be causing you anxiety. Refer to the sections on relaxation and creative visualization in chapter 8, and incorporate some of these practices into your life on a regular basis, especially during stressful times. Take up an activity such as yoga or tai chi.

- Learning which foods to emphasize and which to avoid can be a step toward a life without outbreaks.

- Identify the processed foods in your diet and replace them with healthful foods. Eat plenty of fresh fruits and vegetables. Natural foods cookbooks are easy to find at major bookstores and health food stores and can be a terrific source of cooking inspiration.

- Arginine and lysine are two of the many amino acids our bodies require as part of our overall protein intake. However, arginine is known to contribute to herpes outbreaks whereas lysine helps to prevent them. Therefore, a diet higher in lysine and lower in arginine is part of a herpes-prevention diet.

- This list does not imply that you should completely avoid all high-arginine foods, but common sense dictates that those foods not essential for health be avoided, such as chocolate and coffee. Whole grains, for example, should be eaten in moderation with a dietary emphasis on high-lysine foods.

- Supplementation of 1000 mg lysine daily can help to prevent herpes outbreaks.

- Use 1,000 milligrams of vitamin C daily for prevention of an outbreak, and 2,000 milligrams daily during an outbreak. Do not exceed this dose during pregnancy.

### High-Arginine Foods 🌿
Reduce these in your diet:

- Brown rice
- Carob
- Chocolate, coffee, and caffeinated teas
- Coconut
- Eggplants
- Garbanzo beans (chickpeas)
- Green peppers
- Mushrooms
- Nuts
- Oats
- Raisins
- Seeds
- Sugar
- Tomatoes
- Wheat

### High-Lysine Foods 🌿
Emphasize these in your diet:

- Beans
- Beef
- Cheese, milk, and yogurt
- Chicken
- Eggs
- Fresh fish
- Fresh vegetables
- Nutritional yeast
- Sprouts

## HERBAL RECOMMENDATIONS 🌿

For the prevention and treatment of herpes, you can take herbs that nourish, tonify, and calm the nerves. (Remember, the nerves are where the virus actually resides in the body.) These herbs have antiviral capacity internally and topically, strengthening immunity, reducing moist heat in the body, and "purifying the blood," as old-time herbalists would say:

- The primary herbs for reducing stress and tonifying the nervous system are the antiviral nervines lemon balm and St. John's wort. Additionally, chamomile, lavender, passionflower, skullcap, and catnip may be included in a formula. Take tinctures in warm water, directly under the tongue, or add to an herbal tea. Average dosage is $1/2$ to 1 teaspoon of any of these (or that amount of a combination), two to three times a day.

- The following remedy has proven consistently effective in my practice for preventing herpes outbreaks during pregnancy. It has immune-enhancing properties as well as antiviral potential, and it reduces dampness and heat in the pelvis. Place $1/2$ ounce each of echinacea root and burdock root in a quart jar; fill the jar with boiling water, cap tightly, and let steep for eight hours. Strain and drink, storing the next day's portion in the refrigerator. You can carry this brew with you in a jar or insulated container. Dosage is 2 cups daily, preferably ½ cup four times a day. You should take this remedy throughout pregnancy if you have regular outbreaks; otherwise, begin taking it if you notice prodromal symptoms and continue until all symptoms are gone. It will reduce the frequency and duration of outbreaks. For every week you take these herbs, take a three-day break (for example, seven days on, three days off) to avoid sensitization to the herbs and therefore decreased effectiveness. To prevent outbreaks toward the time of birth, take regularly throughout the third trimester (with the recommended breaks).

- Echinacea and burdock can also be taken in tincture form: 30 drops of each taken four times daily in place of the infusion, following the same recommended course as above. Spearmint can be added for flavor.

- You can effectively treat herpes blisters, reducing discomfort and speeding healing, with several antiviral herbs. A simple combination of licorice root and St. John's wort tinctures can be very effective and can be applied regularly to the sores using a fresh cotton swab. Both of these herbs are specific for the treatment of herpes virus.

- A tincture of calendula oil can be dabbed onto the affected areas with a cotton ball or swab; St. John's wort oil can be dabbed on the affected area during the prodromal phase; propolis tincture can quickly heal oozing sores and reduce pain topically.

- Take sitz baths made with a strong infusion of equal parts of burdock root, echinacea, calendula, comfrey root, and myrrh; steep 2 ounces of dried herbs per quart of water, for four hours.

- In a recent study, significant improvement of symptoms and accelerated scabbing of sores in herpes patients has been shown with the topical application of an extract of lemon balm. Though the preparation was highly concentrated, you may find it beneficial to add this herb to sitz baths and to dab extracts of lemon balm onto the affected area. As it is both relaxing and potentially antiviral, you may want to add a few tablespoons of the dried herb or a handful of the fresh leaves to your burdock and echinacea infusion. To be effective, the study concluded, the treatment must begin during the early stages of infection.

These recommendations are also applicable for oral (type 1) herpes (cold sores). Herpes is spread through skin contact; careful hygiene is essential if you have either type and are caring for a newborn. Up to six months of age, babies are highly susceptible to the herpes virus, with up to a 50 percent fatality rate.

> CAUTION: If a baby shows any signs of illness when there is a family member with either a history of herpes or active herpes, seek immediate medical care for the baby.

# High Blood Pressure

There are two kinds of high blood pressure: high blood pressure that preexists pregnancy and pregnancy-induced hypertension (PIH), which usually shows up after twenty weeks' gestation. Both can compromise the adequate blood flow to the baby, increasing the risks of low birth-weight and stillbirth, and, because of the force of the blood behind the placenta, the risk of a placental abruption, a situation in which the placenta prematurely separates from the uterine wall, a potentially dangerous situation for mother and baby.

High blood pressure in pregnancy can also herald the serious complications of preeclampsia and eclampsia. All women with hypertension in pregnancy should be seen by a qualified midwife or physician.

## GENERAL AND DIETARY RECOMMENDATIONS

- If you are pregnant and have hypertension, work with a nutritionist or physician who can help you to evaluate and improve your diet.

- Prevention is key and is best done with optimal diet and adequate folate or folic acid intake. Some women will need up to 1 to 4 grams of active folate (methylfolate) daily, especially if they have an elevated homocystein level or are positive for changes in the MTHFR gene—which can be checked by your midwife or doctor. This is discussed in chapter 5, What to Eat When You're Pregnant.

- High salt intake has long been associated with the development of high blood pressure in both pregnant women and the general population. In addition, pregnant women have long been told to reduce their salt intake to prevent water retention. However, a great deal of contemporary research has shown that inadequate salt intake during pregnancy can be dangerous, contributing to the development of both high blood pressure and edema. This is because salt helps keep blood volume adequately expanded, which is essential during pregnancy. Lack of salt causes the blood volume to contract, thus the heart must work harder to circulate less blood volume, and the blood vessels also constrict, leading to higher blood pressure. You do need adequate amounts of salt during pregnancy. The key is what type of salt you are getting. Regular table salt, which is used in most prepackaged foods, fast foods, and as table salt, is high in chlorine as well as stabilizers, and sometimes even sugar, and can contribute to high blood pressure.

*Beth began experiencing elevated blood pressure—from an initial reading of 106/60 to a steady 128/74. She began a program of motherwort and hawthorn extract, as well as reducing her work load and increasing her fluid intake. Her blood pressure did not continue to rise and stabilized at an average of 124/68.*

- The key is to lightly salt your foods using sea salt, tamari (natural soy sauce), or earth salt, available at health food stores and in many supermarkets. Cut down on oversalted packaged goods and fast foods, and eat freshly prepared vegetables. In the summertime, you may need to replace extra salt lost through perspiration by salting your food to taste.

- A tasty and nutritious salty condiment that my family has used for years is called *gomasio*, a mixture of sesame seeds and salt (*goma* means "sesame"; *sio*, "salt"). It is said that the combination makes salt more usable by the body's cells. To prepare it, simply roast about a cup of raw, unhulled sesame seeds in a skillet on low heat until they begin to "pop" and turn light brown. Stir continuously to avoid burning the seeds. Just before they are done, add 1 tablespoon of sea salt and stir for a minute more. When slightly cool, grind in a blender or in a traditional Japanese mortar and pestle called a *suribachi* (available at many Asian grocery stores) until the mix is mostly ground but not powdered. Gomasio can be sprinkled liberally on grains, beans, cooked vegetables, and salads. It can be kept unrefrigerated for up to two weeks but is best used within a week.

- Drink plenty of fluid throughout the day. One way I remember to drink enough fluid is to place a full half-gallon jug of water on my table each morning and drink as close to all of it as I can by that evening. You can use the water to make herbal tea as well, and you can drink other fluids such as broths and freshly made fruit or vegetable juices to count toward that half gallon.

- Insufficient intake of essential fatty acids (EFAs) in the diet is also associated with hypertension. It may be improved by adding walnut oil or safflower oil to raw salads and other dishes in place of oils high in saturated fats. EFAs help enlarge blood vessels, thereby reducing high blood pressure. Fatty, deepwater fish such as salmon are high in EFAs. You can supplement your diet with 1 tablespoon of raw flaxseed oil added to a daily salad (do not cook the oil as heat destroys the EFAs). Or take two 500 milligrams capsules of evening primrose or black currant seed oil daily.

- Raw olive oil is associated with low levels of heart disease in Italian women who use it on a daily basis. In Germany, an extract made from the leaves of the olive tree is used to treat essential hypertension. Although the leaves are not appropriate for use during pregnancy, the addition of raw olive oil to the diet on a daily basis may be beneficial for women with high blood pressure (and may work as a preventative). Rather than sautéed vegetables or fried rice, you may want to prepare simple steamed veggies dressed with olive oil and other seasonings.

- A practical way to use raw garlic is to keep on hand a batch of garlic oil for seasoning your foods. Simply peel and mince a whole bulb and place it in a jar with 1 cup of olive oil. Let stand on your counter or in the refrigerator for a couple of days before beginning to use it once a day, garlic and all, on top of salad, beans, pasta, or whole wheat bread. Bread spread with olive oil and garlic is a delicious traditional accompaniment to Italian meals.

- Daily exercise helps to improve circulatory functioning and therefore is an essential part of any program to reduce high blood pressure. A brisk walk

### Foods for Blood Pressure Reduction 🌿

- Ingest 2 tablespoons of olive oil a day
- Use onions and garlic in cooking, salad dressings, and salads
- Drink 2 ounces of unsweetened pomegranate juice a day, diluted in 8 ounces water (or in carbonated water as a spritzer!)

for twenty minutes, working out on a stationary bicycle, swimming, or any exercise that you like that stimulates your circulation is excellent.

- As important as exercise is, the time set aside each day for relaxation, stress reduction, meditation, and the like is essential. This is what I alternately call my sacred time, my sanctuary time, my retreat time, or simply taking space. It is a time devoted to unwinding, letting go of worries and worldly concerns, finding a peaceful place within yourself, feeling centered, breathing deeply, and letting go of physical tension. Occasionally, if you are able, include a full body massage from a professional massage therapist, your mate, or a close friend. This deep relaxation experience is particularly effective if it directly follows your exercise time or a yoga session. Your body's restlessness is reduced from the activity you've just done, and your blood circulation and oxygenation are at a peak, which actually promotes deep rest. (Can you remember how well you slept when you played outside all day?) Refer to chapter 8 for further suggestions on relaxation and creative visualization.

- Taking twenty minutes or so to rest on your left side can help reduce blood pressure because it eases the effort of your heart and circulatory system. This is an excellent position during labor if you already have elevated blood pressure.

- Be honest with yourself, your midwife, or other care provider about your anxieties. This is very important, simply because the effort of damping down your anxieties can contribute to high blood pressure. For example, I once worked with a couple who intellectually seemed to want to have a home birth, but who, on a lot of levels, seemed very afraid of birth. Despite my efforts to help them address their anxieties, they insisted that they were comfortable with birth and wanted to have the baby at home. When the woman finally went into labor, a couple of weeks past due, her blood pressure rose dramatically. We chose to go to the hospital for the birth, where her blood pressure normalized upon arrival. When I mentioned this phenomenon to the attending nurse-midwife, the head of a large midwifery teaching program at a well-known university, she confirmed it, remarking that women can and do psychologically create symptoms that land them in the hospital if that is where they truly feel safer. In our culture, where a technologically advanced birth is considered to be the safest, we cannot dismiss high blood pressure as merely a "psychological factor."

- Blood pressure should be checked at a prenatal visit only after you have had a chance to take your coat off and relax rather than when you first come in. Incidentally, make sure your blood pressure is checked with the appropriate size cuff, as a cuff that is too tight will cause your blood pressure to appear high.

- Funny movies are great for stress reduction!

## HERBAL RECOMMENDATIONS

- When a rise in blood pressure is related to stress and anxiety, herbs may help. These include teas of lemon balm, chamomile, lavender, skullcap, and passionflower. Drink a tea of any of these herbs alone or in combination twice a day to prevent high blood pressure, or sip up to a quart throughout the day to reduce elevated blood pressure. Many of these herbs can also be used as tinctures (although lemon balm and chamomile are best as teas) at a general dosage of $1/2$ to 1 teaspoon taken two to four times a day.

- An excellent herbal combination for the reduction of tension and mild hypertension is equal parts of the tinctures of cramp bark, hawthorn (berries, leaves, and flowers), black cohosh and motherwort. Cramp bark eases physical stress by reducing muscular and nervous tension; hawthorn is a cardiotonic that dilates peripheral blood vessels and improves cardiac output and reduces strain on the heart, thereby reducing blood pressure; black cohosh relaxes the nerves and the muscles and dilates the peripheral blood vessels; motherwort, a gentle antispasmodic and nervine, reduces muscular tension and emotional stress—it contains bitter glycosides that have hypotensive properties, that is, they help reduce blood pressure. This combination can be taken as a tincture beginning after the first trimester.

# Hyperemesis Gravidarum

This is a condition in which you are vomiting excessively and unable to keep much of anything down, causing you to lose vital nutrients and fluids and to become physically exhausted and emotionally drained. If severe, it can become a life-threatening medical emergency in which you become clinically dehydrated with a mineral and electrolyte imbalance; it can also contribute to miscarriage. Treatment requires hospitalization, usually intravenous fluids to replace fluids, electrolytes, and nutrients, as well as medication to control vomiting.

You must seek medical treatment for this condition, but you may be able to mitigate its severity with home treatment, preventing the problem from becoming serious. The following combination of therapies may help you avoid serious illness. It may take a few days to notice complete improvement, but you should see significant improvement within the first twenty-four hours. If you find no relief from these suggestions or if your condition worsens, seek medical care immediately.

## GENERAL RECOMMENDATIONS

Follow all of the general recommendations under "Morning Sickness" in this chapter.

## DIETARY RECOMMENDATIONS

- Each time you throw up, drink a small amount of fluid. In addition, do this throughout the day. Even a quarter cup of liquid every fifteen to thirty minutes can help replace vital fluids. Also, try to eat a small portion of food after you vomit, to prevent clinical starvation.

- To keep your electrolytes in balance, drink 3rd Wind, Gatorade, or Recharge. Or, preferably, prepare the Rehydration Drink by the quart and sip it throughout the day, up to every five minutes. Even if you vomit it up, you will still get some, and over the course of a few hours it will often decrease the frequency of vomiting. This preparation is used worldwide as a remedy to prevent and offset dehydration and electrolyte imbalance, even in cases of severe vomiting and diarrhea in impoverished countries.

- If you are vomiting and unable to keep nourishment down, a nutritive enema is an effective method for infusing nutrients and fluids that can't be tolerated by mouth. This is an excellent technique that I've seen work several times. It can prevent the need for intravenous fluids in a hospital. To prepare the enema, mix 2 tablespoons of blackstrap molasses in 2 cups of warm spring water, and put the solution into your enema bag or bottle. Lying on your left side or on your hands and knees with your chest near the floor, slowly take the enema. If you are quite dehydrated, you may actually retain all the fluid; it will have been absorbed. This can be done up to twice a day during the acute phase of vomiting.

## HERBAL RECOMMENDATIONS

- Take 20 to 40 drops of wild yam tincture, repeated up to every two hours throughout the day, and, in addition, sip ginger tea throughout the day. Try a few of the other herbal suggestions as well.

- A remarkably effective treatment for vomiting is to apply a warm salty pack to your stomach (not over your belly—just directly over your stomach). To do this, heat $1/2$ cup of sea salt in a skillet for three minutes. Put the salt into a pillowcase—it will be very hot. Fold the pillowcase (or other suitable sack) into a small square or rectangular "pad" and apply. If it is too hot, wrap the pad in a towel before applying. This Japanese treatment sends penetrating warmth into the stomach, decreasing spasms and cold, and reducing the frequency of vomiting. Do it when you feel a bout of vomiting coming on, or if you have been vomiting repeatedly.

### Rehydration Drink

- 1 quart water
- Juice of 1 lemon
- 1 to 2 tablespoons honey
- $1/4$ teaspoon salt
- $1/4$ teaspoon baking soda

You can replace the water and lemon with a half quart each of water and orange juice, if you prefer.

# Indigestion and Heartburn

Indigestion and heartburn (burping, gas, occasional stomach upset) are common in pregnancy for a couple of reasons. The increased level of progesterone that softens smooth muscles also slows digestion and sometimes causes incomplete closure of the valve in the upper portion of the stomach, making stomach acid reflux more likely. This is more common in women who are already prone to digestive complaints. The baby's growing size also puts great upward pressure on the stomach. Sensible eating habits and gently soothing herbs usually reduce these problems, as will foods and herbs that help stimulate digestion. Do not use over-the-counter antacids or baking soda: these are generally contraindicated during pregnancy (one exception is the oral rehydration drink).

## GENERAL RECOMMENDATIONS

- Because the dietary recommendations (given below) are the most important part of this approach, follow all those that are relevant to you.

- If lying down causes heartburn, sleep with extra pillows under your head.

- Deep relaxation exercises (see chapter 8) before bed may also allay nighttime heartburn.

- Physical symptoms are sometimes a manifestation of psychic and emotional imbalance. You might take a look at what's "burning you up" or what you just can't digest in your daily life. Do you feel overwhelmed or angry? This is a good time to deal with any issues that are blocking the free flow of your energy. Writing out issues that are weighing on you is a good way to take stock. You may come up with ways to lighten your burdens.

## DIETARY RECOMMENDATIONS

- Oily, heavy, rich, and spicy foods that are hard to digest are major heartburn culprits. Avoid foods that aggravate you, especially at your evening meal.

- Eat small, frequent snacks rather than large meals. A large amount of food consumed at one time can sit in your stomach and disagree with you.

- Have supper at least two hours before you go to bed, and eat a light snack if you are hungry late in the evening. Yogurt is a traditional heartburn remedy.

- To improve digestive activity, try to eat slowly, taking time to enjoy your food thoroughly.

- Some women find that drinking liquids with their meals aggravates them; for others, a glass of water during the meal or a cup of grapefruit juice just before the meal aids digestion. Try it both ways to see what works for you.

- A substance in raw almonds (cyanogenic glycoside) increases the activity of the parasympathetic nervous system, which in turn increases vagal tone (a response of one of your nerves, known as the vagus nerve), slows the heart rate, and improves digestion. A small handful as a snack or after a meal will do the trick. Chew them slowly. Raw cashews may have a similar action.

- A baked potato is sometimes helpful. With a pat of butter or a small amount of cheese and a bit of salt, it makes an excellent snack or small meal.

## HERBAL RECOMMENDATIONS

- Slippery elm bark is wonderful for relieving heartburn. It is best taken on a regular basis or during a bout of heartburn. The easiest way to use slippery elm is to purchase Thayers Slippery Elm Lozenges from a health food store. They are completely safe to use freely during pregnancy, so purchase several packages and keep one in your handbag and one on your bedside table. They have a plain, slightly maple syrup–like flavor and are amazingly effective for reducing heartburn. Suck two to four lozenges per dose, and take up to three doses daily.

- You can also make your own slippery elm lozenges. (See sidebar on opposite page.)

  **CAUTION: Avoid any lozenges that contain coltsfoot or comfrey root while you are pregnant.**

- As an alternative, you can make slippery elm tea. Stir 1 level teaspoon of the herb into a cup of boiling water or warm milk; add a teaspoon of honey and a pinch of cinnamon.

- According to Ayurvedic medicine, an ancient Indian system of medicine, there are three *humors*, or elemental influences in the body: *kapha*, the fluid substance; *pitta*, fire; and *vata*, wind. It is said that too much vata in the intestines causes nervous difficulties. Interestingly, herbs that can be used to reduce "wind" in Ayurvedic terms can also reduce general digestive complaints. Prepare and drink Digestion Tea (see sidebar below) after a meal, or take it before bedtime to ease your digestion.

- Dandelion is an excellent bitter tonic that pregnant women can use for indigestion. Take twenty drops of tincture four times a day or when you are having a spell of heartburn.

### Slippery Elm Lozenges

Take ¼ cup of slippery elm powder and mix with enough honey to make a dough that is neither dry nor sticky. For additional flavor, add 2 to 5 drops of peppermint oil, lemon oil, or vanilla flavoring. Dust a small cutting board with some extra powder. Now roll your dough in this powder to form a long, thin roll (like a snake made out of modeling clay). Next, cut the roll into small pieces the size of a pea or slightly larger. Roll these into little balls and place on a cookie sheet and bake at 250°F for about an hour. When done, these are great to suck on for indigestion (and sore throats).

### Digestion Tea

In a teapot, place ½ teaspoon each of the following:

- catnip or lemon balm
- chamomile
- spearmint
- fennel or anise seeds

Pour 2 cups of boiling water over the herbs, cover the pot, and let it steep for ten minutes. Strain, sweeten with 1 teaspoon of honey, and drink warm.

# Insomnia and Anxiety

Insomnia is a common problem during pregnancy. It can be difficult to go to sleep, and if you have to get up to urinate or if the baby's movements wake you up, you may find it hard to go back to sleep. This section provides you with suggestions for treating insomnia as well as techniques you can use to relieve your anxieties.

## GENERAL RECOMMENDATIONS

- Try to give yourself some wind-down time in the evenings before you go to bed. If you are pushing yourself all day, your body cannot be expected to suddenly switch gears. Instead, induce your body and mind into a quieter state by slowing down your activity level in the evening, reducing stimulating influences (television, phone calls, the computer, the newspaper). Read a pleasant book, take a bath or a walk, read poetry or a story to your children; by slowing down, you will be closer to the relaxed state needed for sleep.

- Regular exercise increases the body's calcium utilization, which in turn helps with relaxation. You will greatly increase your ability to sleep if you practice mild aerobic exercise at least three times per week, for twenty minutes each time.

## DIETARY RECOMMENDATIONS

- One of the most common reasons for insomnia is hunger. You may feel restless, hypersensitive to touch, and slightly nauseated. Perhaps you may even have a vague sense of hunger but are too tired to fix a snack. If this is the case, your problem may be simple to resolve: eat a high-protein snack before bed, especially one that is also calcium rich.

- For some women (myself included), you may occasionally need to eat again when you wake in the middle of the night. You can ask your mate to get up and get a snack for you. Or you can anticipate hunger and keep a snack beside your bed: a cup of yogurt, a banana, a handful of almonds, almond butter on toast or crackers, even a cup of soup—anything nourishing and filling.

- Calcium and magnesium increase relaxation and can be helpful in treating insomnia as well as getting the muscles to relax. Take a supplement with a 2:1 ratio of calcium to magnesium, in the range of 800:400 milligrams, or 600:300 milligrams, before bed each night. Caffeinated foods, coffee, chocolate, and soda can interfere with calcium absorption because they bind to calcium receptor sites in the body.

- Plants that are high in oxalic acid, such as beets and spinach, should be eaten in moderation, not more than once or twice weekly. This is because in high amounts, regular consumption of oxalic acid can lead to kidney stones.

## HERBAL RECOMMENDATIONS

- Herbal nervines are relaxing to the nervous system and mildly sedating; some are calcium rich. They can be used to help you sleep.

- Chronic insomnia may indicate underlying worries and nutritional deficiencies, so you should address these possibilities by improving your diet and exploring your concerns even while using nervines.

- Chamomile tea, or any of the previously mentioned relaxing blends, can be taken before bed to promote sleep. If drinking tea before sleep just makes you have to wake up to urinate—which would be counterproductive!—use a tincture.

- Passionflower is a highly reliable herb to safely promote sleep during pregnancy.

- Milky oat tincture is another nutrient-rich herb that you can use on a regular basis. Used over time, it will help reduce nervous tension. It is best prepared as an infusion rather than as a tea.

- Skullcap, a gentle nerve tonic, promotes restfulness, stress reduction, and sleep. I prefer to use it in tincture form, about 15 drops at a time, but it can be prepared as a tea or in infusions. You can take it up to four times a day during periods of acute stress or twice before bedtime with a fifteen-minute interval between doses. Skullcap tincture can be added to chamomile tea.

*Stacy was having insomnia, nightmares, occasional heart palpitations, and feelings of being overheated. She began taking tinctures of motherwort and skullcap in lemon balm tea several times each day. Within a week, her nightmares and palpitations had ceased, and her feelings of being overheated subsided. She was no longer experiencing insomnia.*

- Lavender blossoms promote a sense of calm. They make a mildly bitter tea that is best steeped for a short time and then sweetened with 1 teaspoon of honey. Use 2 teaspoons of the herb to 1 cup boiling water and steep with a cover on the cup for ten minutes. My own favorite is to use equal parts of lavender and chamomile blossoms to make a tea, add 10 drops of skullcap tincture, and drink hot.

- Other relaxing herbs include lemon balm, catnip, and valerian.

- Herbal baths help you sleep. Create a nightly bedtime ritual: a cup of your favorite relaxing tea to drink, quiet music, perhaps a candle, and a warm bath. To the bath, add 1 quart of lavender or chamomile infusion or 5 to 10 drops of lavender essential oil. Soak for a while, feeling the baby's movements in your womb, and consciously relaxing your muscles. Let the water ease your tension away. (Take care not to fall asleep in the bath, and take fire-safety precautions if you use a candle.)

- For more relaxation techniques to reduce anxiety, refer to chapter 8.

### Chamomile Tea

To prepare, steep 1 tablespoon of chamomile blossoms in 1 cup boiling water for ten minutes; cover the cup while steeping to preserve the volatile oils.

## Itchiness and Skin Troubles

Many women notice that their skin improves during pregnancy. However, you may notice some itchiness. The skin stretches over the belly, breasts, and thighs; extra sweating and decreased bowel functioning cause the skin to work harder in eliminating toxins. The liver, which must now process an increased hormonal load, may be overworked and cause the skin to itch. With a natural diet and herbs, you can prevent as well as reduce skin discomfort during pregnancy. Itching can also be related to stress or signal that something is "getting under your skin." Take a look at whether you are manifesting stress as a skin problem.

> **WARNING: If itching is persistent or progressively worsening, seek medical evaluation. Although rare, it can be a sign of liver disorders specific to pregnancy.**

## GENERAL RECOMMENDATIONS

- Clean your skin with a mild natural soap or just a warm cloth with no soap. Be certain that the soap you use has no additives and no strong perfume. A loofah sponge or a soft body brush can stimulate circulation and clean away dead cells, leaving your skin cleaner and softer.

- Daily exercise gets your circulation moving, bringing a healthy glow to your skin. As your circulation improves, so will your bowel functioning, reducing the burden of elimination on your skin, and the resultant itching.

## DIETARY RECOMMENDATIONS

- Eat plenty of fresh fruit and vegetables daily, as well as whole grains, nuts, seeds, and beans. Eliminate processed foods and reduce your intake of saturated fats, butter, and fried foods.

- Drink a lot of water. About a half gallon a day is ideal for most pregnant women.

- You will have to work on promoting healthy bowel functioning as part of clearing up skin complaints. See "Constipation" (in this chapter).

- Make sure you have adequate essential fatty acids in your diet. Supplement with 1,500 milligrams of a combination of omega-3 acids from fish oil daily.

# Leg Cramps and Restless Legs

Iron deficiency anemia and low magnesium can both cause leg cramps and restless legs as can electrolyte imbalances from excessive perspiration or dehydration. Lack of exercise can also contribute to leg cramps. Cramps and restless legs both tend to be most annoying at night. Improve your mineral intake, get appropriate amounts of exercise, and learn to release tension in your muscles consciously.

## GENERAL RECOMMENDATIONS

- When you get a leg cramp, stand up and place your feet flat and firmly against the floor, as if you are pushing your heels into the ground; then massage the cramped area vigorously and firmly. Another method is to flex your foot gently by holding onto it, curling your toes up toward your knee, and massaging your calf. This can be done while either standing or lying down. If you have varicose veins in that area, don't massage it.

- Avoid pointing your toes during pregnancy—it can start a cramp.

- Exercise daily by walking and doing leg exercises such as leg lifts and lunges. If at all possible, swim or exercise your legs in a pool of water.

- Elevate your legs periodically, preferably for twenty minutes a day, to improve circulation. You can put your feet up on a chair or lie down and put them up on two pillows.

- Stay well hydrated and replace electrolytes if you have been heavily perspiring.

## DIETARY RECOMMENDATIONS

- Increase your intake of magnesium-rich foods (See chapter 5, What to Eat When You're Pregnant) and supplement with up to 800 milligrams of magnesium citrate or magnesium glycinate each evening before bed.

Have your midwife or doctor check your hemoglobin, hematocrit, and ferritin levels to make sure you do not have iron deficiency anemia—if you do, treat it appropriately.

## HERBAL RECOMMENDATIONS

- Herbal foot baths can relieve muscular tension. Soak your feet (and calves, if possible) in a very warm bath to which you add 5 drops of wintergreen oil, 2 drops of camphor oil, and 2 tablespoons of ginger juice. (Grate about a 2-inch section of fresh ginger root and squeeze until the juice comes from it.)

- Foot and leg massage promotes muscular relaxation, improved circulation, and the release of nutrients stored in the muscles, all of which make it useful as a preventative as well as first aid for leg cramps.

The optimal time for a deep foot and leg massage is at bedtime, but it can be given anytime. Use massage oil that contains arnica, St. John's wort, and chamomile, or use a Chinese herbal liniment such as Dit Dat Jiao (see below), an old remedy used for martial arts injuries (credit for this recipe goes to Michael and Lesley Tierra).

- Black haw or cramp bark tincture can be taken to reduce leg spasms. Take 1/4 to 1/2 teaspoon of either herb as needed, up to four times a day. In addition, drink teas or use tinctures made from any of these herbs: chamomile, lemon balm, catnip, lavender, and skullcap.

CAUTION: Persistent leg pain, especially when accompanied by local heat or varicosities (swelling), can be due to phlebitis and merits the attention of an experienced health practitioner. If you suspect this problem, do not massage the area.

*Neesa was having severe leg cramps during the night. She began taking a calcium and magnesium supplement, and within a few days, the cramps ceased. She continued the supplement throughout her pregnancy and had no further problems with cramps.* ◀◀◀

## Dit Dat Jiao ◀◀◀

- 6 parts angelica root
- 6 parts comfrey root
- 4 parts cinnamon bark
- 4 parts valerian root
- 3 parts hyssop
- 3 parts safflower petals
- 3 parts calendula blossoms

Place the herbs in a wide-mouth jar and cover with 80- to 100-proof liquor (I use vodka) until the liquid rises 2 inches over the herbs. Cover the jar, store in a warm, dark place, and shake the jar daily for two weeks. Strain and bottle for use. It warms the skin, dissolves clots and congestion, stimulates circulation, soothes, and heals. Be aware that it may stain fabrics.

CAUTION: This liniment is absolutely for external use only and should be labeled clearly.

# Miscarriage

Miscarriages—pregnancies that end spontaneously—usually before twenty-eight weeks' gestation, occur in about 20 percent of all pregnancies in the United States. Each year in the United States between 600,000 and 800,000 women miscarry. Many women miscarry very early in pregnancy, without ever realizing they were pregnant, having what appears to be a heavy period. Miscarriage rates are highest for young teenagers and middle-aged women (especially when pregnancy has been accomplished with the use of reproductive technologies), and they are more common in early pregnancy than after the first trimester. For women who want to be pregnant, particularly those with a history of repeated miscarriage, losing the pregnancy and the baby is a devastating experience. Many women fear that something is wrong with them as women or that they did something to harm the baby. Because of our culture's refusal to talk about miscarriage, few women know what to do or what to expect when it happens.

If you are experiencing cramping and/or bleeding because of a threatened miscarriage, you can do a number of things to prevent the miscarriage from becoming inevitable if the baby is healthy. The recommendations that follow are in no way harmful to the baby if the baby is otherwise healthy. As blunt as this may sound, miscarriage is nature's way of preventing unhealthy babies from being carried full term. This is painful to accept, but it may spare the baby a life full of adversity. Our bodies have a wisdom of their own. It is important to realize that attempts to prevent miscarriage will not be effective if the baby is not healthy.

Other causes of miscarriage include hormonal imbalances, cervical looseness (called an *incompetent cervix* in the medical world—I detest this term), infections, and nutritional deficiencies. Many of these conditions can be improved naturally.

## PREVENTING A THREATENED MISCARRIAGE

A miscarriage is threatened when you experience spotting, bleeding, or cramping, often with a low backache. These symptoms may begin abruptly or slowly and will usually persist for hours or even days. You may experience some spotting or bleeding and that turns out to be the end of the whole episode, or the symptoms may be so severe you will fear you are going to lose the baby. At this time, the cervix will be closed, but an internal exam is best avoided as it is unnecessarily intrusive and may stimulate the uterus further. Chances are you will still feel pregnant, with continuing breast tenderness and nausea, but you may feel anxious and question whether you are really feeling these signs or you just want to feel them. Most often, if you still feel pregnant, then you are. Usually at about ten to twelve weeks, the baby's heartbeat can be heard with the Doppler—hearing your baby's heartbeat is reassuring and confirms that you have not miscarried though it does not mean that the pregnancy isn't threatened. A midwife can do this test at home. Of course, if the Doppler is tried earlier, the heartbeat may not yet be audible and this could unnecessarily discourage the mother. An ultrasound can also confirm the baby's wellness or indicate otherwise.

## GENERAL RECOMMENDATIONS

- You may have to come to terms with whether in your heart of hearts you really want to be pregnant or whether you or your partner have fears, anxieties, or ambivalence about having a baby. We can influence our receptivity to a baby in our wombs. In no way does this mean that all miscarriages are a result of ambivalence, because the baby's health certainly influences its ability to maintain life. But your desire to continue the pregnancy will support your efforts.

- On a spiritual level, you can communicate your desire to have the baby, also giving the baby permission to go if he or she needs to. Both partners can place their hands on the mother's belly, directly over the womb, and speak to the baby, either aloud or silently. Let your hearts flow with your feelings of love for the baby and for each other, particularly if there is strain between you. Your bond as a couple can strengthen the bond between you and the baby and can aid your efforts to arrest a miscarriage. This can be a strong time of healing.

- As part of making clear your intention for the baby to stay, you can set up a small pregnancy altar in your home on the top of a dresser or bed table or even on a sunny windowsill. You can go to this special place to send loving thoughts to your baby and visualize your womb surrounded with protection. On this altar, place objects that remind you of healthy babies, healthy pregnant mothers, and families: pictures, small statues or figurines, a healthy plant, a stone egg, candles, or anything else that arises from your imagination.

- Treat yourself with the utmost love and care. This is a trying experience that may also challenge your faith in your body. Try to love your body, and don't blame yourself for miscarrying.

- Take time to visualize the baby as healthy, your placenta as strongly connected to your uterus, and your body providing love and nourishment to the baby. Avoid lifting heavy objects and abstain from sexual activity until all signs of miscarriage have been gone for a week. Think positively and use relaxation techniques to help you rest and to reduce anxiety-ridden thoughts. Bed rest *IS NOT* recommended—it does not reduce the risk of miscarriage and can increase your risk of developing clots!

- Warm baths (not hot) can reduce uterine irritability and bring some relief to low backache. A warm bath is also a great place for relaxing and having a good cry to release pent-up feelings.

## DIETARY RECOMMENDATIONS

- In traditional Chinese medicine, it is considered very important to avoid all cold-natured and cold-temperature foods, including foods that have just come out of the refrigerator; cold or iced beverages; fruit and vegetable juices; all tropical fruits, including citrus (unless you live in an environment where they are grown locally); and all foods out of season, including fresh salads when locally grown produce is not available.

- It follows that it is preferable to eat foods of a warmer and nourishing nature, such as soups. Miso soup, prepared from a protein-rich paste of aged soybeans, is excellent, as are chicken soup and bean soups. Also emphasize whole-grain stews and hot cereals, root vegetables, and dark greens until your symptoms have been gone for at least a week. Warm tea or water at room temperature can be taken as a beverage.

- Vitamin E (alpha-tocopherol) has been said to strengthen the placental attachment to the uterus, thereby reducing spotting and the likelihood of miscarriage. It should be taken in doses of up to 800 IU each day for up to three weeks. However, prolonged use may result in the placenta becoming abnormally attached to the uterine wall, a complication in itself. Therefore, do not exceed this dosage, and do not take vitamin E for longer than three weeks. If you have heart disease, do not exceed 50 IU per day without discussing it with your physician.

- Vitamin C plus a bioflavonoid complex—that is, along with the whole group of vitamins that naturally occur with vitamin C in foods—strengthen the capillary bed of the uterine lining, reducing the likelihood of miscarriage. You can take up to 1,000 milligrams daily, including the amount that is in your prenatal multiple vitamin. High doses of vitamin C—in excess of 2,000 milligrams—can cause a miscarriage, so do not exceed the recommended amount.

- Be certain that you are getting adequate protein, carbohydrates, vitamins, minerals, and fluids. Thoroughly read the sections on nutrition in chapter 5.

## HERBAL RECOMMENDATIONS

- Miscarriage Prevention Tincture (page 214) seems to be so effective in preventing miscarriage that midwives across the nation recommend it in one formulation or another. Variations on the theme follow here.

- Partridge berry tones the uterus while also causing uterine relaxation, reducing cramps and contractions. It also supports the nervous system, perhaps helping to reduce the anxiety and apprehension associated with a threatened miscarriage.

- Cramp bark and black haw have very similar actions on the uterine muscles, relaxing them and reducing the severity of contractions. They also have some relaxing effects on the nervous system, making them appropriate choices in a formula for preventing miscarriage. One herb may be substituted for the other, or the two may be used together.

- Chasteberry helps to increase progesterone levels so that the pregnancy can be sustained, most probably by causing the pituitary gland to increase the progesterone levels so necessary for the maintenance of pregnancy. Dose is 1 measured teaspoon each morning throughout the first trimester.

*Marley had been having aching in her bones all night, had dark puffy circles under her eyes, and had vomited in the morning. She had no appetite, severe leg cramps, pelvic pressure, aching in her lower back beneath her ribs, and a temperature (oral) of 99.2°F. She was thirty weeks pregnant (third baby) and was having mild, irregular contractions. She began taking echinacea at a high dose, along with an infusion of uva ursi, increased fluids, vitamin C, and cranberry juice. Within twenty-four hours, all symptoms subsided, and there was no recurrence. Marley gave birth at home at forty weeks' gestation.*

### Miscarriage Prevention Tincture ⫷

- 1 ounce each of tinctures of partridge berry, cramp bark or black haw, and wild yam
- $^1/_2$ ounce of dried ginger root

Dose is 30 to 60 drops every thirty minutes to two hours, depending on the frequency and intensity of cramps, until they quiet down, up to $^1/_2$ ounce of total tincture in one day.

If you have a history of miscarriage, use this formula for at least two weeks past the latest weeks of pregnancy when a previous miscarriage occurred (i.e., if a previous miscarriage occurred at eight weeks' gestation, stay on the formula until ten weeks' gestation). For current symptoms of miscarriage, continue on the formula for one week past the end of the symptoms, taking 45 drops three times daily.

## IF MISCARRIAGE CONTINUES

Not every miscarriage can be stopped. My heart goes out to those of you whose baby is unable to stay with you right now. It is my hope that you will find peace and inner strength in this experience and not blame yourself.

When a miscarriage is inevitable, the bleeding and cramping will not stop until all the products of conception (the tissue that was the developing fetus, the placenta, and the uterine lining that is shed) pass from your body. If the pregnancy ends in the first couple of weeks, it will seem like a normal to heavy period. The further advanced the pregnancy, the more noticeable will be the signs of miscarriage and the more effort you will need to make to clear everything out. Inevitable miscarriage can be suspected when cramping becomes more intense and inconsistent, and the bleeding becomes heavier, to the point of soaking through your clothing or pads. At this time, the cervix will usually be dilating, will be shorter than usual, or will be slightly bulging. It is not necessary for you to check your cervix—I offer this information to those who are familiar with how their cervix feels.

How you choose to handle a miscarriage is a very personal decision. Most women who allow nature to take its course and who receive support through the process will miscarry with no complications. However, miscarriage should not be taken lightly, carrying as it does risks of hemorrhage and infection. The follow-up procedure at the hospital is generally a dilation and curettage, which carries the risk of damaging the womb, or a vacuum suction. Any time you enter the hospital, you are exposed to a host of pathogenic germs unlikely to be encountered in most homes. Also, certain exams and interventions are routine in hospitals. Each woman and each situation must be evaluated on an individual basis and with an open mind, common sense, and a healthy dose of caution.

Your vitality and coherence as well as how long and how much you've been bleeding are good indications of how you are doing. If you feel very weak, strange, or spaced out, or have been cramping heavily (experiencing strong pain, much more than a normal period) and bleeding steadily for more than two hours without emptying the contents of your womb, then going to the hospital is probably warranted. If you are having a lot of cramping but are not bleeding heavily, you can probably continue to take a wait-and-see attitude until you complete the miscarriage or unless bleeding becomes heavy.

> **WARNING: If at any time you become spaced out, fuzzy, incoherent, unusually anxious, sleepy, clammy, or begin to look pale, you need to get to the hospital immediately. These can be signs of shock, which is life threatening.**

If everything seems normal and you choose to stay at home, or if you are unable to reach medical services, the following information will often help to complete a miscarriage at home. Again, if at any time you notice the above signs, seek emergency medical care.

A miscarriage is similar to any birth in that the uterus, in the effort to empty its contents, goes through contractions that build in intensity until it completes the process. However, a normal miscarriage tends to have more continuous bleeding than a normal birth. Women who are miscarrying have not yet experienced the blood volume expansion that usually occurs at about twenty weeks, and therefore are not protected against blood loss. The amount of bleeding in a miscarriage can vary from mild to severe, and, depending upon a woman's health reserves, can make her very weak from blood loss.

Therefore, if you are miscarrying, you should not remain alone. Always have with you someone who can get you to the hospital—and stay in close contact with someone who is knowledgeable about the process, such as a midwife or nurse-practitioner.

At some point during the process, you will pass the tissue that was the fetus as well as the placenta and the sac of membranes that surrounded the fetus. Since you will also be passing clots, you will want to save any such matter for a closer look, in order to determine if you have in fact emptied your womb. A womb not fully cleared out predisposes you to continued bleeding, cramps, and the risk of serious infection. You can look at the tissue yourself (it can be fished out of the toilet if necessary) and try to determine if you see any tissue that looks like a small sac (ranging from about the size of the bowl of a teaspoon to the bowl of a tablespoon, depending upon how early in the first trimester you are). It will be milky white or clear, with some light pink tinges. Clots are more like gelled masses of blood, with some stringiness from the clotting factors that cause the blood to bind. You may find other matter as well, such as small vesicles that look like grapes—a sign that a baby never developed after conception. **(This requires medical attention.)** Saving any material that you pass for analysis by your midwife or physician can help you and them determine whether the miscarriage was complete.

A miscarriage may build up for several days or even weeks before it is complete, with cramping and spotting building in intensity. The actual miscarriage, with regular cramping and heavier bleeding, usually takes place within a couple of hours. After the tissue has been passed, cramping and bleeding will subside, though you may have some more contracting and will definitely bleed some afterward. This will be about the length of time of a regular period, about five days. Heavy bleeding at any time (soaking a pad within thirty minutes is very heavy bleeding) or bleeding persisting for more than five days may mean that pieces of tissue are retained in the uterus. Until the womb is emptied, it cannot completely clamp down, hence the continued cramping is an effort to do so, and the bleeding is a sign that something is preventing this from happening.

> WARNING: Retained tissue can cause serious, life-threatening infection. If natural treatment recommendations (below) for completing a miscarriage are not effective in the first days after the miscarriage, or if at any time your temperature becomes elevated or you notice a foul-smelling vaginal discharge, you should seek immediate medical help.

In some cases a D & C (dilation and curettage) is the best recourse. Sometimes a physician can simply prescribe Methergine (an ergot-rye fungus derivative), used historically by midwives but now available only by prescription. An antibiotic may be warranted if infection is present.

## GENERAL RECOMMENDATIONS

- Have an experienced or a very responsible person with you at all times until your miscarriage is definitely completed. A miscarriage is completed when bleeding and cramping stop and the uterus has passed the products of conception.

- Take it very easy throughout the miscarriage, but do not go to sleep if you are bleeding—drowsiness can be a signal of shock.

- Drink fluids regularly, a cup of liquid every one to two hours, to keep your blood volume expanded. Rehydration Drink (see page 200) can keep your electrolytes and minerals in balance, as can such drinks as Recharge, 3rd Wind, and Gatorade.

- Remember to urinate regularly; a full bladder can aggravate cramping and prevent effective emptying of the uterus.

- Keep yourself warm and comfortable.

- Visualize your cramps effectively emptying your womb. Surround your uterus with light, and imagine the placental tissue releasing from your uterine wall and from your body.

- Have somebody massage your feet or your lower back, especially applying firm pressure to the area over your sacrum. A hot-water bottle applied to this area can also be comforting.

- As painful as this is for you emotionally and physically, try to remember that your body knows how to do this job. Listen to what your body is telling you.

## HERBAL RECOMMENDATIONS

Herbs can be used to encourage complete emptying of the uterus, prevent hemorrhage and infection, help reduce anxiety during the process, and promote healing afterward. Before using herbs, it is essential to have definitive confirmation that the baby is no longer alive. You'd be amazed at how much women can bleed and cramp and still have a completely healthy pregnancy. **Get ultrasound confirmation before using these herbs.** Further, these herbs are not recommended for deliberately stimulating an herbal abortion—they do not work well if there is a viable fetus and can be toxic to a healthy baby.

- Perhaps the most widely recommended herbs for facilitating a miscarriage are blue and black cohosh. Additionally, cotton root bark is excellent and reliable for safely, gently, and effectively promoting contractions. Combined, these three herbs help regulate uterine contractions, reducing spastic muscle contraction and promoting an effective labor. Black cohosh is also an effective nervine, reducing anxiety as well as physical tension. During a miscarriage, tinctures are the most effective and convenient form for taking these herbs.

  To use: Combine 1 ounce each of cotton root and black cohosh tinctures and $\frac{1}{2}$ ounce of blue cohosh tincture.

  **Day 1** Take 1 teaspoon of the above combination every four hours. Discontinue.

  **Day 2** Take 1 teaspoon of the above combination every hour for four hours. Then take $\frac{1}{2}$ teaspoon of the tincture every thirty minutes for four hours. Discontinue.

  Then take $\frac{1}{2}$ teaspoon of the tincture every thirty minutes for four hours. Discontinue.

  Uterine contractions will usually ensue by the end of the second day, if they have not already. They sometimes ensue several hours after the herbs have been discontinued, so don't be discouraged if they do not occur immediately.

  If after two days of using the herbs no contractions begin, skip a day and then resume, following all of day 2 one more time.

- A combination of bayberry bark, shepherd's purse, and witch hazel in the form of tinctures or infusions can be taken to prevent or offset heavy bleeding after a miscarriage. Combine equal parts of the tinctures and take $\frac{1}{2}$ teaspoon every hour if there is mild to moderate bleeding.

  **WARNING: Herbal remedies may help prevent excessive bleeding but are not a substitute for medical care during hemorrhage. If there is heavy bleeding, obtain medical care immediately.**

- Beth root is another excellent herb for promoting uterine contractions and reducing bleeding. It may be added in equal parts to the above formula, or it can be taken on its own, $1/4$ to $1/2$ teaspoon of tincture every two hours to promote contraction or as often as every fifteen minutes during the acute stage of the miscarriage if there is bleeding.

- You can sip a tea of basil or cinnamon throughout and after the miscarriage to promote contractions and prevent excessive bleeding. Steep 1 teaspoon of either herb in 1 cup of boiling water (cover while steeping) for ten minutes.

- If the miscarriage is proceeding efficiently and the main problem seems to be anxiety, sip tea of chamomile and lavender blossoms (2 teaspoons of herbs combined in equal parts to 1 cup boiling water, steeped covered for ten minutes).

## AFTER A MISCARRIAGE

When the miscarriage is complete, your immediate concerns are infection and bleeding. Much healing needs to occur in the first weeks, and then a longer-term physical healing over the following months. For some women, the emotional healing can take years. When you miscarry, your body must make a hormonal adjustment from a pregnant to a nonpregnant state, and you must make an adjustment in your view of yourself. It is important that you give yourself the time to treat yourself gently during the transition. Essentially, you have gone through a birth without getting a baby.

During the first few days after your miscarriage, you can expect to bleed as if you have your period, and you may pass some small clots.

> WARNING: If after four or five days you are still bleeding, or if at any time you are soaking a medium-size sanitary pad in thirty minutes, you must seek immediate medical attention. Also, if you are passing large clots, have a lot of cramping, or notice any foul-smelling discharge, you probably have retained tissue and might have an infection; you will need prompt medical attention.

After a miscarriage, it is advisable to use herbs that work to prevent infection, facilitate the discharge of retained tissue, and promote the healing of your uterus. A general program for the first three days after miscarriage is as follows:

- Check your temperature three to four times each day. It should be normal (close to or at 98.6°F).

- Get plenty of rest, eat nourishing foods such as hearty soups and stews, and drink plenty of fluids. If you have lost a considerable amount of blood, refer to "Anemia" above.

- Take 1,000 milligrams of vitamin C over the course of each day as a preventative measure against infection.

- Take 1 teaspoon of echinacea tincture four times daily to stimulate your immune response and as a preventative against infection. Other herbs that can be used in conjunction with echinacea to prevent infection include calendula tincture (10 drops with each dose of echinacea) or goldenseal tincture (10 drops with each dose of echinacea) or capsules (2 "00" capsules four times daily). Both calendula and goldenseal also promote uterine contractions and act as astringents to prevent hemorrhage.

- Angelica has a reputation for helping to clear the uterus of any retained fragments and is also a warming uterine tonic. Take 15 to 20 drops three times daily to ensure complete uterine emptying, and increase that dosage to as frequently as every two hours if you are having cramps and are passing clots.

- Ground ivy is another tincture with this reputation, and, though I've not used it for these purposes, herbalist Susun Weed recommends it highly for retained placenta after birth. Do not use it to prevent miscarriage, but if you are still cramping and passing clots, take 20 to 30 drops of fresh ground ivy tincture every two to three hours.

- Change your menstrual pad every couple of hours to avoid infection from bacteria in the pad. Be sure to wipe from front to back after you have a bowel movement to prevent rectal bacteria from entering the vulva and causing infection.

- Refrain from all sexual activity until the bleeding has completely stopped. If anyone needs to examine you (your midwife or doctor) make sure that he or she does so with sterile hands. Do not take a bath (you can shower) for the first few days.

- It is essential that you seek a trusted person to help you work out your grief, disappointment, and guilt.

- While you cannot use any substances, including herbs, to heal your grief, a few herbs can help you steady your emotions. If you are unable to rest, you can drink warm teas of chamomile and lavender combined, adding, if you wish, up to 20 drops of motherwort, hops, or skullcap tincture (or a combination of these to equal $\frac{1}{2}$ to 1 teaspoon total). You can also take these as tinctures up to three times a day. Other herbs that support the nerves and promote gentle relaxation include oatstraw, rosemary, lemon balm, catnip, and valerian.

- After the first week, you will probably begin to feel more like your prepregnant self, with all signs of pregnancy gone, particularly if the miscarriage was early. Herbs that nourish the female reproductive system, including those that help to regulate the hormones and the menstrual cycle, can be used to assist you in this transition: red clover leaves and blossoms, red raspberry leaves, chasteberry, false unicorn root, wild yam, calendula, dong quai, ginseng, and licorice. A small amount of ginger root or cinnamon bark can be added to infusions to facilitate the actions of the herbs, while also warming your pelvic region and promoting healthy circulation.

- Chinese herb formulas such as Tang Gui and peony can be used to restore strength and build the blood if there has been much blood loss. Recommendations for anemia can be followed, particularly taking beef stew and using Iron Tonic Syrup, if there is weakness from blood loss.

- This is naturally a painful time for many women, especially if this was your first pregnancy or if you have a history of miscarriage. People who are unaware that you miscarried may ask how the pregnancy is going. You will have to adjust your view of the future, which recently included the expectation of a baby. Miscarriage can also add stress to your relationship with your mate. At the time most women miscarry, the pregnancy may not have felt "real" to the father. He may not take your emotional response to the miscarriage seriously, saying that you can simply try again. For many women, these responses are, at the least, insensitive. The idea of trying again and possibly experiencing such disappointment again is unbearable. For the sake of the relationship, the dad needs to be deeply sensitive to and supportive of his partner. He must listen to you and offer love without dismissing your pain. If you are both deeply grieved and disappointed, this can be a time of holding each other closely and reaffirming your commitment to being a family. If this miscarriage makes the relationship more difficult or intensifies or makes more apparent the stresses you were already having, you may want to consult a professional to help both of you work through the crisis together.

## Women's Nourishment Tea

Mix together $1/2$ ounce each of red raspberry leaf, nettle leaf, strawberry leaf, dandelion root, spearmint leaf, and skullcap, and $1/8$ ounce of ginger root. Store this dry mixture in an airtight jar or plastic bag. To prepare the tea, place $1/2$ ounce of the mixture in a jar, add 2 cups boiling water, and let it steep for two hours. Strain and drink $1/4$ to $1/2$ cup of this brew three to four times a day for six weeks after the miscarriage.

## PREVENTING FUTURE MISCARRIAGES

After having miscarried once, many women are eager to conceive, yet fearful of miscarrying again. In the vast majority of cases, repeated miscarriage is not likely, but it is best to wait until you've had at least three regular periods in a row before you conceive again. By doing so, you allow your uterus to regenerate fully at the implantation site and replenish your blood supply if you bled a lot during the miscarriage. The delay will allow you to experience your next pregnancy as a fresh experience. It really is better not to try to fill the void of your lost pregnancy with another one, but to heal your loss and then embrace your new experience. Books and support groups can assist you in integrating your miscarriage into the experience of your life.

Whether or not you went into your previous pregnancy well prepared, now is a time for getting yourself into excellent health. Creating a pregnancy altar, for example, can give you a place to affirm your desire to have a healthy pregnancy and a healthy baby. The work of creating a gift for your baby, such as a quilt, can give you a concrete way to manifest your intention. Taking 1 to 4 grams of active folate (methylfolate) may help to prevent future miscarriages in women with the MTHFR gene polymorphism. A complete medical workup for blood clotting and immune issues such as antiphospholipid syndrome can help explain the underlying reason for miscarriage.

## HERBAL RECOMMENDATIONS

If you decide that you do want to become pregnant again, you can use herbs to support the pregnancy and prevent miscarriage.

- These are basically the same herbs used to prevent a threatened miscarriage and may be taken both before you conceive (begin taking them up to a month before you try) and then into your first trimester, preferably until two or three weeks after the time of your last miscarriage or throughout the whole first trimester.

- This is the basic formula: 1 ounce each of wild yam, partridge berry, and 1/2 ounce of cramp bark or black haw; 1/4 ounce of red raspberry leaf. Combine all of these herbs and store in an airtight jar or plastic bag. Place 4 to 6 tablespoons of the mixture in a quart jar, fill with boiling water, and steep until the tea is cool enough to drink. Strain out the herbs and drink 1/4 cup four times daily.

- If you find it difficult to prepare or carry these herbs with you each day, use tinctures. Mix together (in a small bottle with a dropper) equal parts of wild yam, partridge berry, false unicorn, and cramp bark, and take 20 drops two to four times daily, the frequency depending upon your miscarriage history. If you've had more than one miscarriage, take the herbs four times daily. Also, if you have such a history, begin taking these herbs for up to two months prior to conception, and consider seeking an experienced doctor of traditional Chinese herbal medicine and acupuncture. The combination of both approaches can be very effective for preventing miscarriage and strengthening you for a healthy pregnancy.

# Morning Sickness

Women experience different degrees of morning sickness ranging from no problem at all to very mild discomfort to nearly constant nausea and vomiting during the first trimester or longer. I once heard it said that the reason it is called "morning sickness" is because it starts in the morning and lasts all day. In actuality, morning sickness can occur at any time of the day or night. Generally, this nausea begins around six weeks into pregnancy and persists until the fourteenth week. It is triggered by different factors:

- Empty stomach, hunger, low blood sugar (hypoglycemia)
- Strong smells (fumes, food cooking)
- Hormonal surges and imbalances
- Normal pregnancy-related changes in the digestive system
- Oily foods
- Very sweet, sugary foods (which, for some women, may include fruits)
- Vitamin or mineral deficiencies
- Lack of exercise
- Fatigue
- Stress
- Constipation
- Ambivalence or anxiety about pregnancy

Nausea that persists much longer than the fourteenth week is usually related to insufficient nutritional intake, unresolved emotional issues, or, rarely, a health problem. If you are experiencing persistent nausea past your first trimester, please seek the help of an experienced health care practitioner who is knowledgeable about the nutritional needs of pregnant women.

There is much speculation as to what actually causes morning sickness and why some women experience it while others don't. Theories include hormonal fluctuations, emotional reactions to pregnancy, nutritional factors, and biological mechanisms that cause women to reject substances that may cause the babies harm. It has been suggested that women who do experience morning sickness have a greater likelihood of a healthy pregnancy and a healthy baby and a decreased incidence of miscarriage. But as yet, no one has come to a definitive conclusion.

Medical attempts to reduce morning sickness through medication have not proven safe for the fetus. The only advice I can give is to avoid eating stuff that prompts nausea and, at the same time, improve your eating habits.

Pregnancy-related nausea is not dangerous, but if you are vomiting excessively, you (and the baby) run the risk of dehydration and severe malnutrition. The condition occasionally requires hospitalization and rehydration with intravenous fluids. (See "Hyperemesis Gravidarum" in this chapter for a further discussion of severe nausea and vomiting during pregnancy.)

## GENERAL RECOMMENDATIONS

- Normal physiological changes of early pregnancy, such as increased levels of estrogen and progesterone, hormones that maintain pregnancy, cause body tissue to become soft and more engorged, and promote such changes as breast enlargement and milk production. They also cause the entire digestive system to slow down and become "softer." The processing of these hormones (equivalent to one hundred birth control pills a day) in addition to these changes can lead to nausea. Moreover, the softening and slowing down of the digestive tract increases the likelihood of constipation, which aggravates nausea; and the incredible amount of work being done by the body causes first-trimester fatigue, which can reduce the likelihood of your eating well, also instigating nausea. By staying well rested, eating well, and taking other precautions to prevent constipation, you can minimize nausea.

- Avoid smells that nauseate you. Don't walk near busy roads if exhaust fumes nauseate you; ask someone to fill your gas tank; let your partner, friends, or relatives help you in the kitchen; and don't prepare those foods that are distasteful to you (by smell, sight, or taste). Often just the smell of a particular food (or a few foods) will completely turn the stomach of a pregnant woman.

- Lack of cardiovascular stimulation—exercise—can contribute to nausea because greater levels of acids and carbon dioxide will build up in the

*Nancy was very nauseated all of the time and was unable to find appetizing, easy-to-digest foods that satisfied her hunger. She'd been a vegetarian for many years, but I had a strong feeling that chicken might settle her stomach and satisfy her. I asked her if she'd consider eating chicken soup, and at this point she was ready to do just about anything. Her husband prepared her a pot of chicken vegetable soup. The chicken broth was immensely satisfying; she ate the meat and vegetables, and began to feel much better. Occasionally, such flexibility can make a tremendous difference in morning sickness.*

blood. A brisk walk in fresh air or some form of exercise daily can reduce the severity of nausea. Regular exercise also reduces fatigue and prevents constipation. Eating a snack about a half hour before you plan to be active will help prevent nausea or low blood sugar. It is also essential that you eat well after exercising to replenish lost calories, particularly if the exercise is strenuous. If exercising triggers nausea, try regular massage, a form of passive exercise.

• You can reduce nausea by getting plenty of rest, using relaxing herbs, and asking for help with your responsibilities if you are fatigued. Perhaps you can think of at least one or two people who will watch your older kids or help with household chores.

• Ambivalence about the pregnancy can cause internal tension that may exacerbate feelings of nausea, and vice versa. Even women who are completely thrilled to be pregnant may have misgivings. It is important to acknowledge and accept your feelings rather than feel guilt for these emotions. Worrying that you are harming your baby with your negative thoughts only adds to your tension. Talk to friends, other pregnant women, or a midwife or counselor; use a journal as an outlet for your concerns. It is perfectly normal to go through a time of uncertainty— children are a great responsibility. Perhaps there are steps you can take to enjoy your pregnancy. If your ambivalence is triggered by the nausea, know that this too shall pass and you will soon begin to enjoy your pregnant body much more.

• *Nei guan* patches or bracelets (for example, Sea-Band) are special devices available from acupuncturists and at many health food stores that put pressure on acupuncture point PC-6. They have been clearly demonstrated in clinical studies to reduce nausea associated with pregnancy. They are completely safe and therefore worth a try.

## DIETARY RECOMMENDATIONS

• Eat small, frequent snacks that contain complex carbohydrates and protein. A simple snack of a cheese sandwich on whole-wheat toast will quell hunger, prevent blood sugar from dropping with ensuing nausea, and is quick and easy to prepare. Other suggestions are tofu sandwiches, bean or chicken noodle soup, pasta dishes, yogurt with granola, peanut butter on toast with a topping you enjoy, hummus on toast, chips, crackers, or vegetable sticks. Eating snacks about every two hours is less likely to trigger nausea and vomiting than a few large meals a day; by eating about every two hours, you prevent your stomach from becoming empty. Eating a snack such as crackers or toast when you first wake in the morning can reduce the nausea caused by stomach acids in an empty stomach. Some women find that a grapefruit or a small cup of fruit juice just before a meal gets the digestive juices going just enough to help food go down. Breakfast, or the lack of it, can set the tone for your entire day, so be sure not to skimp on it.

- Many women wake in the night and find themselves unable to return to sleep. This is frequently due to unrecognized hunger; the baby takes nourishment from you even while you sleep, causing you to become hungry at odd hours. Try eating a snack before bed and, if necessary, in the middle of the night. This may seem odd, but you'll find yourself sleeping more restfully. Yogurt makes an excellent before-bed or middle-of-the-night snack, as does toast, a banana, a handful of almonds, or any food that you enjoy and that digests easily.

- Always carry nutritious food with you whenever you go out. Skipping food for as little as two hours during early pregnancy can cause you to feel extremely nauseated and depleted. Hypoglycemia—low blood sugar—can trigger not only nausea but also dizziness, headaches, hot flashes followed by cold sweats, anxiety, and fainting. A mix of nuts and seeds, a container of yogurt, or small containers of other food can keep you feeling well. Don't tide yourself over with caffeinated beverages or candy bars—you won't be providing yourself or your baby with any nutrients, and you'll still end up feeling nauseated in the long run. There is no need to feel embarrassed about eating in public wherever you are, even if no one else is eating.

- Many pregnant women find that drinking fluids aggravates nausea, but actually dehydration causes worse problems. You need to drink plenty of liquids throughout the day. If you are vomiting, you are losing fluids; you must replenish them. Water with a squeeze of lemon, natural grape juice, grapefruit or orange juice, or carbonated water with a squeeze of lemon are all choices that may be palatable and can help settle your stomach. Avoid coffee, soda, and other caffeinated or sugar-laden drinks. Taking sips of liquids throughout the day may be easier than drinking glassfuls at a time.

- Oily foods are hard to digest. Sweet foods may lead to a quick blood sugar drop after an initial energy boost, leaving you feeling nauseated and drained. Choose foods that are prepared by steaming, water-sautéing, or baking; and choose foods that contain complex carbohydrates. These will sustain your energy level in a more balanced way and are also easier to digest, helping you avoid nausea. See chapter 5 for a discussion on nutrition.

- Nutritional deficiencies—too little iron, vitamin B-complex, magnesium, or calcium—as well as too little protein or complex carbohydrates can cause morning sickness. Perhaps you didn't really notice these deficiencies until your body had the increased nutritional demands of pregnancy. Consider taking a vitamin and mineral supplement designed for pregnant and lactating women. See chapter 5 for more information.

- Unfortunately, supplements may aggravate nausea in the first trimester. If this is the case, avoid taking supplements on an empty stomach; instead, try taking them while eating. Some women have found that taking between 50 and 200 milligrams of vitamin $B_6$ daily can alleviate nausea because it helps regulate blood sugar levels. This is safe. Once you have gotten past the nausea stage, you should take vitamin B-complex, not just $B_6$ by itself.

- Another remedy is to take 50 milligrams of vitamin K once daily, and 250 milligrams of vitamin C twice daily.

- Talk with your midwife or physician about taking betaine HCL and digestive enzymes—both can dramatically improve your digestion and reduce nausea.

## HERBAL RECOMMENDATIONS

During my pregnancies, I would try something for nausea and that would work for a few days. But I would quickly become tired of a certain herb and keep changing. Play around with different approaches to see what works for you.

- Ginger is by far the best-studied herb for the treatment of nausea and vomiting in pregnancy, having been demonstrated effective in numerous clinical trials. It can improve sluggish digestion and gently warms the digestive tract. It is pleasant tasting when sweetened lightly with honey.

Steep 1 teaspoon of freshly grated ginger root in 1 cup of boiling water for ten minutes and sip throughout the day, not exceeding 2 full cups daily. Or take 2 "00" capsules of powdered ginger every few hours, but do not exceed ten capsules per day. Sucking ginger-flavored hard candies or crystallized ginger can also be helpful. Look for these in a health food store.

- Dandelion root is one of my favorite herbs. A bitter herb, it promotes digestion, calms and strengthens the stomach, improves the appetite, and supports the liver, which must work overtime during pregnancy to process the increased quantity of hormones surging through you. All of these functions of dandelion root plus its safety during pregnancy make it an excellent choice for addressing morning sickness either alone or in combination with other herbs, such as ginger root. To prepare an infusion, use 4 to 6 tablespoons of the dried roots or twice that amount of the fresh roots in 1 quart of boiling water, and steep for four hours. Strain and take a few mouthfuls at a time, up to 2 cups daily. Or take 30 drops of tincture three or four times a day.

- Chamomile tea is another of my personal favorites. It relaxes the stomach, reduces acidic feelings, supports the liver, and improves appetite. It also reduces anxiety and tension. Prepare by steeping 1 tablespoon of the herb in 1 cup of boiling water for ten to fifteen minutes. Cover while steeping to retain the volatile oils in the blossoms. You can sip it throughout the day or drink up to 2 cups daily.

- Wild yam is an herb that reduces irritation and irritability in the hollow organs, including the stomach and the uterus. It is an excellent herb for reducing nausea, relieving vomiting, and relieving spasms in the stomach. The dosage is up to 30 drops, 4 to 6 times daily. Combined with dandelion root (30 drops of each), it has proven very effective for reduction of nausea and vomiting.

These are other remedies that can be useful for morning sickness:

- Ginger ale or carbonated lemon water, plain or to which you add 20 drops each of ginger root tincture and dandelion root tincture.

- *Umeboshi* (sour plum) candies, available at natural food stores (the sweet-and-sour taste of umeboshi can allay nausea).

- In addition, some women gain relief from acupuncture or acupressure treatment.

# Preeclampsia

Preeclampsia, formally called *metabolic eclampsia of pregnancy*, is a serious and potentially life-threatening condition that can arise late in pregnancy. The consequences include placental insufficiency (insufficient nutrients get to the baby, resulting in undernourishment and low birth weight), placental abruption (the placenta separates prematurely, which predisposes the mother to hemorrhage and is often fatal for the baby), premature birth, complicated birth, and, if untreated, eclampsia, a complicated stage of the disease that can lead to seizures and liver damage for the mother, and even her death. In short, it is not a condition to be ignored or taken lightly, and if it develops, it absolutely requires medical treatment in the hospital.

> WARNING: Any pregnant woman with a severe headache, upper abdominal pain, or high blood pressure should be evaluated for preeclampsia. It usually develops late in pregnancy but can arise in the early postpartum period as well.

The causes of eclampsia are related to a few factors, including heredity, faulty implantation of the placenta, and poor nutrition. Following a healthy diet and lifestyle during pregnancy should, in itself, be preventative. Women with a mutation in the gene for MTHFR may be at increased risk and may benefit from the addition of a supplement of 1 to 4 grams of active folate (methylfolate) early in pregnancy.

## DIETARY RECOMMENDATIONS

- Take 1 to 4 grams of active folate (methylfolate) daily.

- Make sure you get between 60 and 100 grams of protein per day. Women who get enough protein rarely develop preeclampsia. (See chapter 5 for a full discussion of protein and nutritional sources.)

- Complex carbohydrates are essential for energy, blood sugar stability, and healthy weight gain. Eat whole-grain foods at all meals and as part of snacks during pregnancy.

- Do not restrict salt.

- Take a daily prenatal vitamin.

- Junk foods are an express ticket to poor health. They keep you from eating nutritious foods because their high sugar or fat content causes you to feel full. Teach yourself about healthy eating. Your health and your baby's health depend upon it!

# Stretch Marks

Silvery jewelry draped on the belly of Woman, adorning her and reflecting her ability to grow and change—this is how I view stretch marks. Some women develop stretch marks; others don't. Various factors may be involved: heredity, nutrition, tissue strength, the elasticity of your skin. There are no definitive answers.

Most women do not want stretch marks any more than they want sagging breasts. Our society tells us that flat bellies, perky breasts, and tight flesh are sexy and beautiful. Unfortunately, these characteristics are present in young women who have not borne children. They are associated with a sexual ideal that few women actually approach, even before childbearing. The body after childbearing is typically not considered beautiful in our culture, although in others, for example the culture of the Mbuti pygmies of Africa, pendulous breasts are respected because they reflect the fact that a woman has nourished her community through her very flesh. In fact, the more a woman's breasts sag, the greater her status in the community. It is time that we, as active participants in our culture, take pride in our individual form, shape, and markings, and help change society with our values.

Women are often advised to massage their bellies with cocoa butter or other oils to prevent stretch marks. This is all well and good. It may be effective, but it is not loving yourself to rub your belly with the intention of preventing stretch marks. To love yourself, rub your belly and breasts with awe at the amazing accommodation your body is giving to your growing baby. Babies can feel this attention, and they love it! Praise and admire yourself, and you will be rewarded with self-respect, whether or not you develop stretch marks.

Oils and herbs that are nourishing for the skin include cocoa butter, pure almond oil or wheat germ oil, shea butter, and herbal oils made with chamomile, orange, lavender, calendula, rose petals, and comfrey. You can make a wonderful belly and breast massage oil by mixing a few handfuls of any of these herbs in a pint jar with 2 cups of an oil of your choice. If you wish to use cocoa butter, use half oil and half cocoa butter, and carefully cook the mixture over a double boiler for twenty to thirty minutes because cocoa butter is hard at room temperature. Cover the jar tightly and let sit on a sunny windowsill for one week. Strain the oil into another jar, and it is ready for use. You can add a few drops of an essential oil for fragrance, if you wish, and 400 IU of vitamin E as a preservative and skin nutrient. See appendix A, Herbal Preparations, for further instructions on making herbal oils.

# Swelling

As pregnancy advances, mild swelling of the feet and ankles is considered normal and does not require medical attention. In late pregnancy, swelling of the face and hands, particularly if it begins suddenly, or is accompanied by severe headache or high blood pressure, can be a sign of preeclampsia and requires immediate medical attention.

## GENERAL RECOMMENDATIONS

- Elevate your feet for twenty minutes, three to four times each day. Put them on pillows to get them above the level of your heart to improve circulation. The weight of your uterus on your blood vessels impedes venous return, causing blood and fluid to collect in your lower body. Allowing this circulation to freely return to your heart not only reduces swelling, but also can be invigorating and lift depression.

- Lying on your left side while you sleep or rest can also improve circulatory function, thereby lessening swelling.

- Exercise for thirty minutes a day. Pelvic rocks, leg lifts, and gentle yoga can enhance circulation and reduce swelling.

## DIETARY RECOMMENDATIONS

- Be certain that your diet contains plentiful amounts of high-quality protein and adequate salt plus all the other nutrients you need.

## HERBAL RECOMMENDATIONS

- Soak your feet in a warm bath (deep enough to cover your feet), using $1/2$ cup of Epsom salts in a basin, or 1 cup in the bathtub. To the Epsom-salted water, you can add lavender flowers, rose petals, sprigs of rosemary, or drops of wintergreen oil.

- Get a regular foot massage. Arnica oil rubbed into swollen areas reduces soreness and aching in muscles and joints. Your mate or friend can easily give you a foot massage as you sit together. Perhaps have your partner rub your feet before you go to sleep at night. (Lie on your left side to enhance effectiveness.)

- Drink a nettle and dandelion leaf infusion, 1 to 2 cups daily, or take $1/2$ teaspoon of each of these tinctures twice a day to improve general circulation, help the kidneys remove and retain the appropriate amounts of fluids for your body, and improve your overall nutritional status.

## Urinary Incontinence

Involuntary leaking of urine (urinary incontinence) can happen when you sneeze, cough, jump, or perform any physical exertion. It can vary in amounts ranging from a small dribble to a deluge wetting your pants. It is a common problem in America. Women who have already borne children are particularly susceptible to developing incontinence because the muscles of the pelvic floor stretch during birth. Further pregnancies will aggravate this tendency because pregnancy increases urination and because the uterus places a great deal of pressure on the bladder. Incontinence is not inevitable, however. In fact, it is quite preventable. Pelvic floor exercises are discussed below.

The *levator ani* is a muscle group, commonly known as the pelvic floor, that forms a sling extending from the back of the pelvis to the front and supports all the pelvic organs and structures, including the uterus, bladder, vagina, urethra, and rectum. When the muscles forming this sling become weakened, they are less able to support these organs, and signs and symptoms of weakness begin to appear; one of the earliest and most common is urinary incontinence. At the first sign of this, do pelvic floor exercises to improve the tone of your muscles. If you wait until you have severe incontinence or prolapse of your organs, you will have to work much harder to improve tone.

- Pelvic floor exercises, generally referred to as *Kegel exercises* after the physician who originally popularized them, are a nonsurgical method of healing urinary incontinence. Chapter 7 offers specific exercises that are beneficial for the prevention and healing of pelvic floor weakness, the symptoms of which include incontinence. Follow these exercises each day.

*Lydia was having mild swelling in her right hand and right foot, as well as heart palpitations. She had no history of heart disease, and the swelling seemed to be associated with sleeping on her right side. She began to sleep on her left side and take a combination of motherwort and hawthorn extracts. Within three weeks the swelling ceased to occur, and the heart palpitations also stopped.* ❦

With commitment, you will see improvement after a few weeks, even if you begin during pregnancy.

- You may wish to try a sitz bath with astringent herbs such as witch hazel and nettle as topical astringents.

# Urinary Tract Infections (UTIs)

The urinary tract consists of the kidneys, ureters, bladder, and urethra. Growing a baby places an additional load on these organs. Hormonal changes that soften the ureters, along with the weight of the womb upon them and the bladder, increase the likelihood of stasis, or stagnation, in your bladder or ureters, which breeds bacteria that can lead to infection.

The medical approach to bladder infections is to automatically treat with an antibiotic, and for women who have no symptoms but have bacteria in their urine, antibiotics are also recommended. Furthermore, for women who have more than two urinary tract infections in pregnancy, preventative antibiotics are recommended daily for the remainder of the pregnancy. The concern is that untreated, there is an increased risk of preterm delivery. Also, pregnant women are more susceptible to serious kidney infections as a result of untreated bladder infections.

Symptoms of a bladder infection include extra-frequent urination (it's normally somewhat frequent during pregnancy), often accompanied by burning or pain ranging from subtle to severe; low abdominal tenderness just above the pubic bone; recurrent Braxton-Hicks contractions (the contractions normally occurring during pregnancy that you may or may not have noticed); flu-like feelings; and, in rare cases, vaginal bleeding. A kidney infection (pyelonephritis) is evidenced by fever, chills, backache, and a worsening of the previously mentioned bladder infection. If you suspect that you have either a bladder or kidney infection, please let your midwife or doctor know right away. Kidney infections in pregnancy do require treatment with antibiotics.

Bladder infections (cystitis) can be treated effectively with botanical therapies. Some women prefer to avoid antibiotics when possible during pregnancy due to emerging reports of possibly increased risks of the later development of inflammatory bowel disease and possible other medical problems when babies are exposed in utero. Some also prefer a more natural approach.

**WARNING: Left untreated, a bladder infection can easily become a kidney infection. Kidney infections can place the mother's health in danger, so the care of an experienced health professional should be sought immediately.**

Refer also to "Vaginal Infections" in this chapter for recommendations. Because the urethra (the entrance to the bladder) is located just above the entrance to the vagina and not far from the rectal opening, bacteria can easily spread to the bladder.

## GENERAL AND DIETARY RECOMMENDATIONS

- Dramatically reduce your intake of all sugars—sugar breeds bacteria.

- Be sure to urinate as soon as you feel the urge, and empty your bladder thoroughly. When you hold urine too long, it can serve as a breeding ground for bacteria. Too many women are accustomed to putting off urinating until they can no longer wait. This is an unnecessary and health-defeating habit based on not listening to our bodies and on making external tasks more important than the body's needs. When you've got to go, go!

## HERBAL RECOMMENDATIONS

- Take echinacea root tincture, 1 drop per every 2 pounds of your body weight every four hours until symptoms are gone and then 20 drops three times a day for a few more days to prevent recurrence. Echinacea is antimicrobial, it is an immune-system tonic, and it reduces inflammation.

- Use uva ursi tea or capsules. Uva ursi is a leathery-leafed bush that provides a medicine known to act on urinary tract infections, working specifically as an antimicrobial and gentle diuretic. It is a highly effective remedy for cystitis.

  Uva ursi contains a chemical constituent called *arbutin* that transforms into another chemical called *hydroquinone*. Hydroquinone is considered toxic, and thus uva ursi should not be used during the first trimester unless under the supervision of a qualified practitioner, and should only be used for short durations (five days or less). Unlike standard antibiotics, the use of uva ursi for UTIs does not lead to recurrent bladder infections, nor does it lead to problems with yeast infections as so often happens with prescription antibiotics.

**WARNING: Any signs of pyelonephritis require medical attention.**

- To prepare uva ursi, place $1/4$ cup of the leaves in a quart jar along with $1/4$ cup of marshmallow root (an herb that is soothing to the urinary tract) and fill the jar with boiling water. Some herbalists say that this herb is more effective when steeped in cold water, and you can certainly do this, but I've found that hot water makes an effective remedy. Either way, remedies directed to the urinary system are most efficient when they are at room temperature or slightly cool—hot herbal teas encourage perspiration, whereas cool teas encourage urination. Let steep for two hours, strain, and use. The dosage is $1/4$ cup every four hours for subtle signs of a UTI, $1/2$ cup every four hours for obvious symptoms, and 1 cup every four hours for a raging UTI. Do this until symptoms abate, decreasing the dosage as symptoms subside, but continuing to take 1 cup a day for five days at the maximum. Although baking soda is generally contraindicated during pregnancy, for chronic UTIs, the effectiveness of the uva ursi may be enhanced by taking 2 "00" capsules of baking soda three times daily.

- Wild yam is a urinary tract antispasmodic, reducing pain and inflammation. Take $1/2$ teaspoon of tincture, two to four times daily, along with the other herbal treatments above if there is bladder pain, spasm, or associated uterine contractions accompanying the infection.

- Take 500 milligrams of vitamin C four times each day for three to five days. Vitamin C encourages acidification of the urine, helping to kill bacteria and is also a reputable resource for helping the body resist and overcome infection.

- Cranberry juice has been clinically demonstrated to be effective as an antimicrobial, preventing bacteria from adhering to the wall of the bladder, thus preventing recurrent UTIs. A product called cranberry D-Mannose, a cranberry extract, is easy to take and very effective for UTI prevention. Eight ounces of unsweetened cranberry juice, can be taken daily as an alternative. I recommend that women start taking it *while* treating the UTI and continuing after for at least two weeks, or throughout the pregnancy if recurrence is a problem. It can also be taken in conjunction with an antibiotic if one is needed.

# Vaginal Infections

Engorgement of the vulva with increased blood circulation and hormonal changes that alter the balance of vaginal acidity cause vaginal infections and heavy mucous discharges, a common complaint of pregnant women.

Some vaginal infections, such as chlamydia and beta-strep, can be asymptomatic (or at least some women may be unaware of the symptoms) yet pose a health threat to a baby born vaginally in the presence of these organisms. For example, chlamydia can lead to respiratory infections and blindness in newborns.

> **WARNING: If you suspect that you have gonorrhea or syphilis, especially evidenced by vaginal or vulvar lesions or discharge, or if you have had a positive test for either of these infections, seek medical treatment as soon as possible—before the birth of your baby. The risks of these diseases outweigh the risks of treatment.**

## GENERAL AND DIETARY RECOMMENDATIONS

- Drink plenty of fluids.

- Wear cotton underwear or none at all. Synthetic fibers trap moisture in the crotch area and provide an excellent breeding medium for many organisms. You may even need to change cotton underwear by midafternoon if it gets damp from discharge or sweat.

- Wear loose-fitting cotton clothing; try not to wear pantyhose, especially those without a cotton panel in the crotch.

- Avoid all concentrated sugars, including honey, maple syrup, and corn syrup.

- Avoid caffeine, including coffee, caffeinated sodas, chocolate, and black tea.

- Don't use bubble bath, bath oils, bath salts, or strongly perfumed soaps in your bath or around your vulva.

- Use white, unscented toilet paper.

- Don't use any "feminine hygiene" or douche products.

- Practice excellent personal hygiene: Wipe from front to back after a bowel movement. Rinse your vaginal area with water (no soap) during the day and then pat dry, to reduce the likelihood of bacterial or fungal growth.

- Bacteria spread readily in heat and moisture. Dry yourself gently but thoroughly after bathing or swimming. Change out of wet swim clothes soon after swimming. Change undergarments and launder (with a mild detergent) frequently. Use 1 cup of white vinegar in the rinse cycle of your washer to remove soap residue, acidify garments, and disinfect and remove any remaining body fluids.

- Don't scratch your crotch. Scratching will further irritate the area and spread the infection or lead to a superimposed bacterial infection, for example, a staph infection.

- Avoid intercourse during the worst symptoms or if painful. Your partner may also need to be treated to prevent reinfecting you. Men can harbor asymptomatic infections that you then pass back and forth, and your attempts at eliminating the infection will be ineffectual.

- Use some form of natural lubrication during intercourse, such as almond or coconut oil.

- Urinate after sex and thoroughly rinse yourself off with warm water.

- Take 500 to 1,000 milligrams of vitamin C complex (with bioflavonoids) daily.

- Eat plenty of live-culture plain yogurt each day to both prevent and treat vaginal infections. This is especially good when you are under stress or when you must take antibiotics. (Let your doctor know if you are prone to yeast infections before you take antibiotics.)

- Cut back on simple carbohydrates (starches and sugars, including processed flour and fruits and fruit juices).

- Eat nutritious meals that emphasize whole grains, vegetables, and high-quality protein foods. Reduce the amount of sweets in your diet while you are treating vaginal infections. Eliminate sweets altogether if you are prone to such infections. This includes reducing the amount of fruit you eat (get your vitamins and minerals from extra vegetables) and using rice, oats, millet, and other whole grains in place of yeasted breads whenever possible. These dietary changes alone can often clear up a yeast infection.

- Reduce stress in your life as much as possible. Get adequate rest. Infections thrive when your body is run-down.

## VAGINAL YEAST INFECTIONS

*Candida albicans* is the fungal organism that causes what is commonly known as a yeast infection. All women have this organism in their bodies, but various circumstances, such as the increased vaginal discharge that accompanies pregnancy (especially if you wear clothes that prevent adequate aeration of your vulva), changes in vaginal pH, increased consumption of carbohydrates, and stress and fatigue, can lead to the overgrowth of yeast. Symptoms of a yeast infection are itching and redness of the genitals; white, thick, yeasty-smelling discharge that may look curdy like cottage cheese (but might be slight); burning of the vulva; and painful intercourse. There may be frequent urination or even an attendant bladder infection caused by irritation of the urethra. Symptoms range from mild to severe, with itching and burning being the most noticeable.

If you have no history of yeast infection, the problem will likely clear up with no treatment at all as soon as the baby is born and can simply be kept under control with simple dietary and herbal treatments. If you have a history of yeast infections, continue treatment after birth if they persist. Occasionally, a woman who has a yeast infection may pass it on to the baby during birth. The baby may then develop oral thrush, which can cause digestive distress, and in turn pass it on to the mother's nipples, causing her mild to extreme discomfort and difficulty with breastfeeding. Therefore, you should at least try to minimize all yeast infections with natural remedies before the birth. For treatment of thrush in babies and on the breasts, refer to my book *Naturally Healthy Babies and Children*.

Treatment of a yeast infection includes close adherence to all the general and dietary guidelines above as well as the following internal remedies and your choice of external applications.

### Internal Remedies

- Take a probiotic daily.

*External Remedies*

Choose a few of these suggestions to see what works best for you. Note that all of these remedies are for external use only.

- Live-culture, plain, unsweetened yogurt is perhaps one of the most effective remedies for treating yeast infections. Applied directly to the vulva, it reduces inflammation, restores your pH balance, and also restores your normal vaginal flora while destroying the yeast. The best method I know for applying the yogurt is as follows:

  1. An hour before you are ready to apply the yogurt, put about ¼ cup of it in a dish and let it come to room temperature. This is merely a comfort measure, but it is well worth it—very cold yogurt applied to your vuvla will certainly cause you to catch your breath! Use a separate dish so you don't inadvertently contaminate the entire yogurt container.

  2. Insert your index finger into your vagina and gently scoop out all the yeast you can. (This is best done in the shower.) Yeast likes to thrive on the vaginal walls and in the area up around the cervix. Do not attempt to scrape it out; merely get out what you can so that the lactobacillus and acidophilus cultures in the yogurt stand a better chance of overcoming the yeast.

  3. Wash your hands thoroughly; then put 1 to 2 tablespoons of the yogurt onto your index and middle fingers. Smear this up inside your vagina.

  4. Now apply the remaining yogurt to your vulva, the external genitals, getting it well into the creases.

  5. Repeat this twice a day during an acute yeast infection, and a couple of times a week if you are prone to yeast outbreaks. You can actually open a couple of your probiotic capsules and add these to the yogurt before applying to fortify the effect of this treatment.

- One traditional remedy for yeast infections is to peel a clove of garlic very carefully so as not to nick it at all. Dip the clove in olive oil and insert vaginally. Remove after several hours or in the morning if you've put it in before bed, which is ideal, as it stays in more easily if you are lying down. Repeat with a fresh clove each night for several days in a row. It may occasionally cause burning, but garlic is highly regarded for its antifungal properties. This treatment is not always effective.

- A combination of calendula, lavender, and thyme can be made into an infusion that can be used as an antifungal rinse (not a douche) for your vulva. To make the infusion, mix 1 ounce of the herb mixture per 4 cups of water; boil for twenty minutes, and then strain. Rinse once a day during an active yeast infection.

- A vaginal probiotic with an applicator is available from Klaire Labs; it is called Ther-Biotic and contains *Lactobacillus reuterii*, which has been shown to be especially helpful in reducing vaginal infections.

- Slippery elm bark powder, marshmallow root powder, and comfrey root powder soothe irritated and inflamed tissue. Sprinkle the powder on your irritated vulva or rinse yourself with a tea of any of these (or a mixture of them), getting some up inside of yourself with your fingers. To prepare a tea for external application, mix 1 tablespoon of herbal powder with 1 cup hot water, stirring well. You can also prepare an infusion with the whole dried herbs (not the herbal powder) by boiling 4 to 6 tablespoons of the herbs in 4 cups of water for twenty minutes.

- The juice of the aloe vera plant is exceptionally cooling and soothing and mildly antiseptic as well. It can be scraped from the inside of fresh leaves or purchased at natural food stores in the form of aloe vera gel and applied. In the case of an extremely irritated vulva, you can spread some of the gel onto a cloth menstrual pad and wear it throughout the day.

- A healing salve can be applied to your sore vulva as a comforting ointment. To prepare, refer to appendix A, Herbal Preparations. Include chickweed, plantain, and calendula in your salve.

- "Yeast•Gard" is a prepackaged homeopathic suppository that many pregnant women find highly effective for the treatment of persistent, difficult yeast infections. It is available at many regular drugstores and even at some supermarkets. Health food stores also carry it.

- You can also create your own *boluses* (suppositories) for persistent yeast infections. While it takes a little effort, they are well worth it, highly effective, and you can make a large supply at one time that keeps indefinitely in the refrigerator if well wrapped. Boluses are effective for soothing inflamed vaginal membranes and are mildly antifungal. Because it is safer not to douche during pregnancy, an herbal bolus is an excellent way to apply herbs up in the vagina. By varying the herbs, you can use boluses after birth to heal hemorrhoids.

To prepare a supply, you will need $1/2$ cup of coconut oil or a combination of coconut oil and cocoa butter in equal parts (these oils become hard when cold, holding their shape, but then soften when warmed) and approximately $1/2$ cup of powdered herbs. A good reliable combination includes equal parts of goldenseal powder, echinacea powder, and slippery elm powder. Melt the oil in a small pot over low heat but do not boil. When the oil is melted, turn off the stove. To this mixture add 2 teaspoons of calendula oil and 7 drops each of lavender essential oil and thyme essential oil.

Add the herbal powders and stir thoroughly until the mixture forms a thick, sticky dough. Add additional powder if necessary. Now put some slippery elm powder onto a cutting board and place your "dough" on it. Roll the dough into the shape of a long, thin log (like the clay "snakes" you made in kindergarten) about as thick as your index finger. Cut the roll into pieces $1^1/2$ to 2 inches in length, wrap in foil, and put into the refrigerator. They will be ready to use in a couple of hours.

To use, place one bolus up into your vagina each night before bed. The bolus will melt and can be a bit messy, so wear underwear with a pad or sleep on a towel. Repeat for a week.

## GROUP B–STREP INFECTION (GBS INFECTION)

Anywhere from 15 to 40 percent of all healthy women at any given time will be carriers of the organism known as beta-hemolytic streptococcus—or in short, beta-strep or group B strep. This organism, which is different from group A strep (which causes sore throats, for example), is also found on the bodies of more than 40 percent of all newborns. Of these newborns, only 1 percent will become ill from this bacteria. Given the prevalence of this germ with the relatively low incidence of related disease, one might wonder why physicians and midwives would be concerned about its presence in a woman's vaginal canal prenatally. The reason is that the rate of complications (including paralysis from meningitis, kidney damage, and sight and hearing loss) and mortality to the baby is very high. It is estimated that as many as two thousand babies in the United States die each year as a result of beta-strep infection.

Because it is simple to determine the presence of vaginal beta-strep with a vaginal culture, many doctors and midwives will request that you have a culture done at around thirty-five weeks pregnancy. If beta-strep is found, then your birth will be handled differently. It is recognized that the risk of beta-strep infection for the baby grows in the presence of prolonged rupture of membranes—that is, the longer your bag of waters has been broken, the greater the risk. The greatest risk is considered to occur when the waters have been ruptured for over twenty-four hours; therefore, part of the management of your labor will be to get your baby to be born before twenty-four hours has passed, even if this necessitates a cesarean. The other aspect of labor management is to place the mother on antibiotics either prior to her due date, at the time the membranes rupture, or when the mother commences labor. Different doctors, hospitals, and midwives will all vary slightly in the length of time they allow a woman to labor before becoming aggressive in speeding along the birth, and their schedule for prescribing antibiotics may also vary.

There are advantages and disadvantages of routine prenatal screening for beta-strep, and there are natural treatment options that can begin to be address the potential for infection well before a woman is due to begin labor. There are also practical and natural approaches to facilitating labor and monitoring the baby during labor and in the immediate postpartum so that aggressive methods are rarely required. Here I will discuss the advantages and disadvantages of routine prenatal screening, as well as natural treatments you might wish to try if you do have vaginal beta-strep.

The primary advantages of prenatal testing for beta-strep are that if the organism is present, you can approach your labor in a way that considers the optimal health of the baby. You can also do things prenatally that reduce the number of organisms, reducing the likelihood of your baby contracting the organism and becoming infected. The main disadvantage is that the standard accepted medical procedures for "managing" pregnant and laboring women with beta-strep can be unnecessarily invasive, especially considering that this organism is a natural part of the vaginal flora for so many women, the vast majority of whom will have babies who don't become infected.

All practitioners who assist pregnant women face a double bind with beta-strep: because of its prevalence and potential risk, it is too dangerous to ignore, but because of the prevalence of the organism and relatively low incidence of problems, it is excessive to assume the worst for all women. Therefore, the best approach may be to identity those women with the greatest risk and to provide natural prenatal treatment to reduce the presence of the organisms.

> **WARNING: Any newborn showing signs of infection should receive immediate medical care.**

Women who are at the greatest risk for having an active beta-strep infection that could be passed on to the baby include those with a history of urinary tract infections and/or persistent yeast infections, who go into labor before thirty-seven weeks, whose bag of waters ruptures prematurely, whose membranes rupture prematurely or before contractions begin, who had a fever before or during labor, who previously had a strep-infected baby, or who had a high beta-strep count earlier in the pregnancy. Not all of these factors prove the presence of beta-strep; however, if these symptoms have occurred and the presence of beta-strep is confirmed, you should try to reduce the bacterial count starting at about thirty-two weeks. If you have been positive for beta-strep, the baby should be monitored carefully in the first few days after birth.

## GENERAL RECOMMENDATIONS

- A positive attitude toward your body, your sexuality, and your pregnancy, along with excellent nutrition, can go a long way in promoting the strength of your immune system and preventing and reducing any infections.

- Visualize your vaginal canal as pink and healthy, a nourishing place that your baby will pass through on his or her birth journey.

- Any vaginal infection, such as yeast, that causes tissue irritation can allow other organisms (such as beta-strep) to attack the damaged tissue. Therefore, follow all of the general recommendations for vaginal organisms found at the beginning of this section (page 237).

- Be informed (read, research, ask questions, and consult your inner wisdom) about the risks, interventions, and issues surrounding beta-strep. Be sure that you understand whether you've had this test performed and what your care provider's protocols are. Some midwives, for example, might not be aware of beta-strep, while others might immediately transport you to the hospital if your waters have been broken for longer than eighteen hours.

- Don't allow yourself to panic when a health care provider is nervous about beta-strep. Remember, while the risk to a small percentage of babies is high, the overall incidence of this infection compared to the incidence of its presence is very low. Do your best to reduce risk factors, but continue to trust your inner guidance regarding yourself and your baby.

- Refer to other relevant topics in this book if you are experiencing factors associated with beta-strep, for example, urinary tract infections.

## DIETARY RECOMMENDATIONS

- Overall, an excellent diet will keep you healthy and prevent organisms from proliferating in your vaginal canal. Refer to chapter 5, What to Eat When You're Pregnant, for a full discussion of this important aspect of your prenatal health.

- A prenatal vitamin and mineral supplement can provide nutrients that may be missing in your diet and can aid your body in creating a healthy environment that prevents a growth of unwanted organisms.

- As beta-strep infections may often occur in conjunction with persistent yeast infections, addressing the dietary factors that cause yeast to proliferate may assist you in reducing beta-strep.

- A probiotic may help keep the colonization of GBS in the colon under control; this is the primary source of colonization to the vagina so may help to reduce the incidence GBS vaginal infection.

## HERBAL RECOMMENDATIONS

Ideally, you will begin treatment at about thirty-two weeks, on confirmation of the presence of beta-strep in a vaginal culture, a urine sample that showed beta-strep, or a rectal sample. (Some doctors will do both a vaginal and rectal swab.) Treatment will include taking herbs orally that strengthen your immune system and applying herbs vaginally that will restore your healthy vaginal flora, that will enable your body to reduce bacterial overgrowth, and also that will directly fight the bacteria. As you enter the last few weeks of pregnancy, from thirty-seven weeks onward (since your baby is unlikely to be premature), most midwives will be willing to assist you at home if this is your plan. In the hospital, your baby will also be considered close to full term and will not be treated as premature in most circumstances. At thirty-seven weeks, you can therefore begin to use certain herbs both orally and vaginally that are sometimes considered labor stimulants, but are nonetheless effective for reducing bacterial infections.

- At thirty-two weeks, begin to take a supplement of 500 milligrams of vitamin C, and 1 cup of burdock root and echinacea root infusion. To prepare the infusion, steep $^1/_2$ ounce of each of these herbs in 4 cups of boiling water for two hours. Strain and take the above dose, storing the rest in the refrigerator for the next day.

- Eat a lot of fresh garlic every day.

- Take $^1/_2$ teaspoon each of echinacea and astragalus tinctures twice daily. You can also get dried astragalus in the herb department of your health food store and cook two strips into a pot of rice or soup two to three times per week. Remove the strips when done cooking and eat the rice or soup. Astragalus is an immune system tonic well known in the Chinese pharmacopoeia, but also grows in America.

- Beginning at thirty-two weeks and continuing until the end of your pregnancy **(Warning: Discontinue if you have broken waters!)**, take regular sitz baths (a bath filled to the height of your hips is sufficient for this) and rinse your vaginal and perineal area with a clean "peri-bottle" (available at a pharmacy or through Cascade HealthCare Products— see Resources) of the following herbal infusion and essential oil mixture.

---

### Garlic Remedies

- Chop a clove of fresh garlic and mix with a teaspoon of honey. Swallow this without chewing it. This can be done several times a day, preferably with a meal.
- Make a garlic elixir by blending $^1/_2$ cup of honey, $^1/_4$ cup of apple cider vinegar, and half a bulb of fresh garlic in your blender until it is fairly liquid. Take $^1/_2$ teaspoon up to twice a day. Adjust the taste as necessary with more or less of the honey or vinegar.
- Chop fresh garlic onto a salad, or mix with olive oil to use as a dressing or dip French bread into this as a condiment.
- Take garlic perles according to the dosage on the brand you purchase.

---

This will help to restore vaginal flora while reducing vaginal bacterial counts. Infuse equal parts of thyme, calendula, rosemary, and yarrow, 6 tablespoons of the herbal mix per quart of water, and steep for thirty minutes. Strain into a clean jar and add ¼ cup of sea salt and 10 drops of lavender essential oil. If you are taking a sitz bath, add the entire jar to the tub; if you are using a peri-bottle, fill the bottle and save the remainder as a refill. You can bathe as often as once daily, and can cleanse your vulva with the peri-bottle solution after each time you urinate. Spreading your labia apart with your fingers makes the peri-rinse more effective.

- After thirty-seven weeks (and if your waters are not broken), you can begin to insert one capsule of goldenseal into your upper vaginal canal each night before bed. Goldenseal is a natural antibiotic. You can ask your midwife or other care provider to show you how to do this if you are uncomfortable trying it on your own, but all you need to do is push the capsule inside of your birth canal as far as you can reach. The capsule will dissolve, releasing the goldenseal. You may want to sleep in an old shirt and put a towel under you to protect the sheets should the goldenseal leak out.

- After thirty-seven weeks, if your care provider agrees, you can use the above peri-bottle and sitz bath rinse as a very gentle douche. It is imperative that the douche be low and gentle, as a forceful douche can cause an embolism in the mother, which can be fatal. If you are uncomfortable with douching, spread your labia wide open, and irrigate your whole vulvar and perineal area quite thoroughly.

Remember that a healthy diet and a healthy sexuality—both your sense of yourself as a sexual being, and your relationship with your partner—are also important in preventing and healing vaginal infections. No amount of herbal remedies can compensate for these aspects of your life. Please give thought to these ideas and find ways to nourish your body as well as finding clarity, joy, and love in your sexual experience. Also, always remember that in healing any infection, you are working to restore your body's natural balance and defenses, not just attacking organisms.

# Varicose Veins and Hemorrhoids

Varicose veins occur when the valves that keep blood flowing one way through the vessels become weak, allowing blood to pool up in the veins and causing the veins to become lax and distended. This weakness of the valves may be due to diet, lack of exercise, or heredity. The hormonal changes of pregnancy can contribute to laxity of the valves. Pregnancy also predisposes women to congestion of blood in the lower body because the pressure from the heavy uterus reduces venous return from the legs and pelvis. Varicosities most commonly occur in the legs and feet, the vulva (vulvar varicosities), and the anus (hemorrhoids). They generally become more pronounced as pregnancy advances. Vulvar varicosities may or may not be noticeable until labor, but women usually notice large ones during pregnancy. A gentle birth and hot compresses applied to the distended veins usually prevent trauma to them. Occasionally, bleeding or a hematoma (an internal pooling of blood from a broken blood vessel) can result and may require medical care. Hemorrhoids usually become enlarged at the birth with the mom's pushing and may persist for a few days postpartum. Again, gentle pushing whenever possible will reduce their severity. Constipation during pregnancy aggravates hemorrhoids and should be treated because it can cause other health problems as well.

Natural remedies regularly taken and applied can effectively prevent and reduce varicose veins.

## GENERAL RECOMMENDATIONS

- Follow all dietary and exercise suggestions, and use appropriate herbal remedies.

- Exercise can vastly improve circulation and must be a vital component in both the prevention and treatment of varicosities. By increasing your circulatory rate, you are effectively removing stagnation in your blood vessels and directly reducing blood congestion, a primary factor in varicosities.

- Take a brisk walk for thirty minutes each day or ride a stationary bicycle for approximately that length of time. Swimming is also an excellent form of exercise—as you swim, feel the water massaging your legs.

- Yoga postures and commonly known exercises such as leg lifts, lunges, and, if you can do them, shoulder stands can successfully strengthen your circulatory system and encourage venous return.

- Vigorous pelvic tilting vastly improves pelvic circulation and venous return. This can be done for five to ten minutes daily. Stand with your feet shoulder-width apart, hands on your hips. Slowly tip your pelvis forward, then backward, gradually increasing your speed until you are swinging your hips forward and backward vigorously. You can also roll and rock your hips and make "figure eights" in belly-dancer fashion.

- Dance, dance, dance! Open to your creative flow as you exercise your legs, pelvis, heart, and spirit.

- In addition to exercising daily, you will want to spend at least twenty minutes, twice a day, with your feet elevated higher than the level of your heart. Putting your legs and feet up on two pillows as you recline is usually sufficient. If you are sitting at a desk, put your feet up on it!

- Don't sit in one place for any length of time because it encourages insufficient pelvic and leg circulation. Get up and walk around about once an hour for ten minutes to improve blood flow. You should do this on long car trips in your third trimester of pregnancy even if you don't have varicosities.

- Use support stockings if you have severe varicosities. If you put them on in the morning when you first get up from bed, they will be easier to get on and the most effective. You can dust a bit of slippery elm powder on your legs to help them slide on.

  **CAUTION: Never massage varicose veins. Massage can dislodge clotted blood and lead to an embolism, a very dangerous situation. If you see signs of phlebitis (swelling, heat, pain, infection around the veins), seek the care of an experienced midwife or physician.**

*Jody had severe leg and vulvar varicose veins that had become very difficult during her second pregnancy. Now in her third pregnancy, the varicosities were becoming a problem, and were looking extremely red and inflamed. She began a therapeutic dietary and herbal program to include foods high in bioflavonoids and rutin, nettle infusion and hawthorn tincture, and regular periods of rest as well as daily inversion on a slant board. Externally she applied compresses of witch hazel extract from the pharmacy. The inflammation completely subsided and while the varicosities were still obviously visible throughout the pregnancy, they remained unproblematic; Jody gave birth at home with no difficulty.*

- Visualizing your varicosities reducing in size may help you produce this result. Imagine your life flowing smoothly as you imagine the blood flowing smoothly through your veins. Let obstructions dissolve, and let yourself feel strong and supported.

## DIETARY RECOMMENDATIONS

- A diet rich in healthful foods, especially a variety of whole grains, high-quality protein, and vegetables, will supply the nutrients you need for the maintenance of a healthy circulatory system.

- Vitamin C with bioflavonoids is vital for maintaining strength in the walls of blood vessels. Foods high in vitamin C include all citrus fruits, rose hips, dark green leafy vegetables, cherries, sprouts, strawberries, cantaloupe, broccoli, tomatoes, and green peppers. In addition, a daily supplement of up to 1,000 milligrams of vitamin C with bioflavonoids can add to the integrity of the circulatory system. Bioflavonoids are brightly colored substances that often appear in foods in conjunction with vitamin C. Sources of bioflavonoids include lemons, grapes, plums, black currants, grapefruit, apricots, buckwheat, cherries, blackberries, and rose hips. In citrus fruits, they are more abundant in the inner skin (the white, pithy part) than in the juice. One of the main purposes of ingesting Vitamin C and bioflavonoids is to increase the strength of the capillaries. One of the bioflavonoids, rutin, is specifically used to treat hemorrhoids and varicose veins and is best taken in conjunction with vitamin C and a bioflavonoid complex. The best way to obtain rutin is to eat foods with a high bioflavonoid content.

- Vitamin B complex is also necessary for healthy veins. Brewer's yeast, fortified nutritional yeast, whole grains, and organ meats contain substantial levels of B vitamins. B vitamins are also produced in our intestines to some degree when we have healthy intestinal flora. Alcohol, sugar, and antibiotics can damage intestinal flora, while an active-culture yogurt, eaten in small amounts on a regular basis, can help replenish and restore intestinal flora. A B-complex supplement can also be taken.

- I cannot overemphasize the importance of including dark leafy green vegetables in the diet on a daily basis. Salad greens, like romaine, green or red leaf, and butter lettuce, as well as greens that are tastier cooked, like kale, collards, and mustard, dandelion, and turnip greens, all promote health and vibrancy and are particularly important for a healthy circulatory system.

- For hemorrhoid prevention, avoid and treat constipation and straining on the toilet!

## HERBAL RECOMMENDATIONS

This section is divided into two parts: herbs to be used internally and those to be used externally.

### Herbs for Internal Use

- The humble but highly nourishing nettle is by far the best herb for pregnant women with varicose veins. Because of its high mineral content and its ability to tonify the blood vessels, nettle makes a wonderful supplement and astringent brew for varicose veins. Women with severe varicosities may find that the blood vessels don't disappear completely, but will not develop into painful and swollen veins. Prepare an infusion using 1 ounce of herb to 1 quart of water, and steep for two hours. Drink between 1 cup and 1 quart daily depending upon the extent and severity of the varicosities.

- Horse-chestnut seed extract is the most widely used herb in Europe for the treatment of varicose veins and is considered safe for use during pregnancy, though safety data is lacking. I recommend it regularly in a dose of 250 to 312.5 milligrams (equivalent to 100 milligrams of aescin, the active ingredient) twice daily.

- A deficiency of essential fatty acids may exacerbate varicose veins, so you may want to take 500 milligrams of one of these oils once a day: evening primrose, flaxseed, black currant, or borage oil.

### Herbs for External Use

- For hemorrhoids, use witch hazel extract from the pharmacy; you can use prepurchased Tuck's pads or make your own with witch hazel extract and cosmetic pads. Alternatively, you can apply horse-chestnut seed extract cream directly to the hemorrhoids twice daily

- Use a topical lidocaine gel if painful or itching.

- For varicose veins also apply witch hazel by soaking wash cloths or kitchen-type towels in the extract from the pharmacy (it's very inexpensive, so purchase a few bottles as time) or apply horse-chestnut seed extract twice daily.

- Dit Dat Jiao liniment, a Chinese herbal liniment intended for martial arts injuries, makes an excellent application for varicose veins. It reduces inflammation and bruising and promotes healthy circulation in the areas to which it is applied. It is most suitable for varicosities of the legs and feet. The recipe for this easy-to-make and worthwhile liniment is found on page 209. It has many applications beyond pregnancy, including for bruises and injuries in which the skin is unbroken and for all muscle aches and tight muscles. Do not apply to hemorrhoids!

  CAUTION: **Do not massage varicose veins.**

# Herbal Preparations

>>>×<<<

*Preparing your own herbal products* is both rewarding and cost-efficient. This section provides you with all of the information you need to begin this venture. In Resources, later in the book, you will find companies that supply herbs and other products, such as jars, oils, and even decorative labels, that are useful in herbal product making. While you do not need fancy equipment or supplies for making or packaging most herbal products, get yourself a sturdy notebook for recording your recipes, successes, and failures, and be prepared to have friends, relatives, and even neighbors putting in requests for that special liniment or salve that you have created!

## Gathering Herbs

Whether you plan to grow your own herbs, gather them from the wild, or purchase them, you are certain to find the process of making your own medicines fun and rewarding. In the long run, putting up a batch of iron tonic or belly massage oil that will last for months is less costly than buying vitamins or lotions. Although you may still need to buy packaged preparations, I think you will find yourself relying more and more on your home remedies. Making your own herbal preparations is empowering, giving you a new understanding of herbs.

### FROM THE WILD
Whenever possible, use herbs harvested from the wild in the area where you live. An uncultivated plant has more vitality than a cultivated one, just as wild animals retain more of their natural qualities than those living in zoos or in houses. Instruction in plant identification and harvesting is beyond the range of this book,

but I encourage you to learn to identify a few local medicinals to enhance your connection with the plant world.

> WARNING: If you are going to use local wild plants, be absolutely certain that your plant identification is accurate. Mistakes can be fatal. Seek the advice of experienced botanists at local nature centers. Never pick plants that grow near roads, under power lines, or in any areas exposed to chemicals including fertilizers, pesticides, or toxic wastes. Choose healthy plants in clean, unpolluted areas.

Don't pick all of the plants in one location. Leave enough growing to repopulate the area. Avoid endangered or rare plant species. Always offer your thanks to the plants and ask for their blessing and assistance in healing.

## FROM YOUR GARDEN

Herb cultivation is a very broad field, one in which I am by no means an expert. I do know, however, that I experience the greatest joy when I am sitting in a garden filled with healing plants. Many herbs are not only useful but also beautiful, particularly when they are in bloom. Then the bees and butterflies will flock to your garden, and you will feel a new, profound connection to the plant world.

When you grow your own herbs, you will develop a greater understanding of them. You will see how they change through the seasons and what conditions cause them to thrive, and you learn to recognize their scent and appearance.

The initial investment in seeds or starter plants can vary. A small well-cared-for garden can provide you with enough herbs to make small amounts of a few remedies. A large garden could potentially provide you with all the herbs you could want and some to spare for friends or for sale. Many herbs are prolific, so even a small plant, tended well, will yield a plentiful harvest over time. Perennials return year after year, so if your budget is limited, go with these instead of annuals. Not at all herbs grow in every climate or location, so consult books and local gardening stores to determine exactly what can be raised where you live.

# Purchasing Herbs

It is preferable to obtain organic, wild-crafted plants or at least organically cultivated plants. Preparations such as capsules and tinctures should likewise be prepared from organic herbs. Many inorganic herbs are fumigated with fungicides and insecticides during storage, and some are even irradiated. Check your sources.

All herbs and herb products should have a fresh smell, and their color should resemble that of the fresh plant. Herb freshness will affect the potency and therefore the effectiveness of your treatments. A moldy, dusty odor indicates that the herbs are not fresh. Look closely for insects; one infested batch of herbs can let tons of bugs loose in your home. They can then get into other herbs in your pantry as well as your food.

# Preparing Herbs

Seeing different herbs turn water, alcohol, and oils into lovely shades of gold, red, orange, green, and brown is nothing short of magic. Preparing one's own remedies adds a special potency to the medicines: that of love and care.

Common supplies are required for making everything from teas to salves in your kitchen: glass jars of varying sizes with lids, glass or stainless steel pots, a sharp knife, a small funnel, a mesh strainer, a vegetable grater, measuring spoons, and a cutting board. Water, vegetable oil, vodka, and beeswax complete the list once you have the herbs you need.

Some preparations cannot be made easily at home. These include essential oils, which require special equipment for extraction, and herbs that must be powdered finely with a special grinder. If you wish, try experimenting with a coffee grinder to see if you achieve a powder that is satisfactory.

If you plan to use your own preparations as primary medicines, you will want to look through this book and plan ahead. Tinctures take weeks to prepare, for example, so you will need to have these on hand, since if you need a tincture today you can't wait. Keep in mind that most herbal preparations such as oils and tinctures will keep for up to a few years (oils must be kept refrigerated), so if you prepare small batches of medicines at a time, you will find that little gets wasted.

Throughout this book, I've made every effort to give specific measurements for preparations in the form of teaspoonfuls, tablespoonfuls, and ounces. For convenience, I sometimes have listed recipe ingredients in parts. You can translate these to any measure you are using. For example, if you are using tablespoons, 1 part would be 1 tablespoon, 2 parts would be 2 tablespoons, and a half part would be about $^1/_2$ tablespoon. Choosing an appropriate measurement for these recipes allows you to determine the amount you want to make.

## FORMS OF PREPARATION

Water, alcohol, and oil are the most common bases used. (*Menstruum* is another word for a base or solvent.) Some herbalists also use vinegar, but since it is not suitable for all herbs, I reserve it for steeping fresh culinary herbs.

### Water Bases

The Earth, plants, and our bodies are primarily made of water, so our bodies accept water-based solutions easily. These include teas, infusions, decoctions, and syrups. Infusions and decoctions are used for baths, washes, and compresses as well as internal use.

**Tea** is the most basic herbal preparation. To make a tea, steep 1 teaspoon to 1 tablespoon of a dried herb in 1 cup boiling water for up to twenty minutes. Herbs with a lot of volatile oil content are easily extracted this way and so should be covered during steeping to prevent loss of their oils. Peppermint, catnip, lemon balm, chamomile, fresh ginger, lavender, and seeds such as fennel and anise are in this category.

**Infusions** are medicinal-strength teas. More herb material is steeped longer in slightly more water than is usual for a tea. The result is a darker, stronger-tasting, more potent brew. Pint- and quart-size canning (Mason) jars are the best vessels in which to make infusions.

To make an infusion, steep 4 to 6 tablespoons of chopped, dried herb or twice that of chopped, fresh herb in either a quart or pint jar filled with boiling water for anywhere from a half hour to eight hours. The steeping time and the amount of water correspond to the intended strength of the remedy and also depend upon the part of the plant being used. The general recommendations are as follows:

- *Roots*: Use 1 ounce dried root to 1 pint of boiling water; steep for eight hours.

- *Bark*: Prepare as for roots.

- *Leaves*: In general, when using delicate leaves or those rich in essential oils, use 1 ounce of dried leaves or 2 ounces of fresh leaves to 1 quart of water and steep for one to two hours. Thick leaves (such as uva ursi) require steeping for up to six hours. Leaves used for nutritional purposes (such as nettle) should be steeped for up to eight hours.

- *Flowers*: As these are delicate, steep 1 ounce of dried flowers in 1 quart of boiling water for a maximum of one hour.

- *Seeds*: In general, you first gently crush the seeds with a mortar and pestle and then steep them for up to thirty minutes. Usually $^1/_4$ to $^1/_2$ ounce of seeds per pint of water is sufficient.

Generally, the dosage of an infusion ranges from $^1/_4$ to 1 cup, two to four times daily. Sometimes an infusion is sipped throughout the day.

**Decoctions** are concentrated infusions. This makes for a strong brew that is taken in smaller dosages. A decoction is an excellent way to take herbs when it is difficult to tolerate large amounts of a strong-tasting preparation. The method is especially suited for nutrient roots such as yellow dock and dandelion because you can get concentrated doses of minerals without having to drink cupfuls of beverage. Leaves, flowers, and seeds are rarely decocted as their constituents can be damaged by boiling.

To prepare a decoction, make an infusion and steep it for up to eight hours. Strain the liquid into a saucepan (discarding the used plant material), and simmer it until it is reduced to between one-quarter and one-half of the original amount. Take care not to boil off all the liquid. Reducing a pint of liquid by one-half (down to a cup) takes approximately an hour. Pour into a glass jar, let cool to room temperature, and then refrigerate.

When unsweetened, decoctions last in the refrigerator for up to three days. Two tablespoons of honey per $^1/_2$ cup of liquid or about 2 tablespoons of brandy per cup of liquid can extend the life of a decoction for up to three months when kept refrigerated.

Dosage is usually 1 teaspoon to 1 tablespoon, two to four times daily.

**Syrups** are easy to make from a decoction. Syrups have two main advantages over decoctions: you will more readily take a small amount of a sweet-flavored medicine than any amount of an unpalatable one; and the large amount of sweetener in the syrup preserves the preparation so that you can keep it in the refrigerator for a longer time than a sweetened decoction. Simply sweeten your decoction by adding an equal amount (by weight) of sweetener. One cup of a decoction is 8 ounces, so a decoction of this amount would require 8 ounces of sweetener. I use $^1/_4$ to $^1/_2$ cup of honey per cup of liquid and find this adequate; honey is considered to be twice as sweet as sugar. Add the sweetener to your hot decoction, bring to the boiling point while stirring, and then immediately pour into clean jars. Cool to room temperature, label, and refrigerate. Dosage is similar to a decoction but of course will vary from herb to herb.

**Herbal baths** are a rejuvenating ritual and are useful for all sorts of complaints: sore muscles, injured skin, exhaustion, irritability, congestion, and fever, to name a few. Be very careful to avoid burns from overly hot water.

- *A foot bath* is given in a basin of water wide enough for the feet and deep enough to reach at least above the ankles. Add a quart of herbal infusion to enough hot water to fill the basin.

- *A sitz bath* requires a quart of decoction or a couple of quarts of infusion placed in a shallow tub with enough water to reach hip level.

- *A full bath* can be made two ways. You can fill a cotton cloth or sock with at least an ounce of herbs and fasten the closed cloth to the faucet so bathwater runs through it while the tub is filling. Squeeze the sack now and then to wring out the tea. This will make a mild but pleasant herbal bath. You can also prepare a couple of quarts of herbal infusion or decoction and then strain these into the tub.

If you keep the door to the bathroom closed, the aroma of the herbs and any volatile oils will fill the air, adding to the relaxing effect of the bath. Herb baths are a nourishing gift to yourself during pregnancy. Floating herb flowers directly in the tub makes for a fun bath, but use a screen of some sort to keep the plant material from clogging the drain.

**Poultices and compresses** are ways of applying herbs externally to specific areas of the body. You can quickly make a poultice by mashing, bruising, or even chewing fresh herbs into a pulpy mass and applying it to the affected area. You can also make one by mashing fresh or dried herbs (dried herbs need to be moistened with warm water first), and spreading the material on a thin cotton cloth, which is then applied to the area. A hot-water bottle can be placed over the herbs or cloth to retain the warmth. Poultices are used for stings, bites, localized infections, wounds, boils, abscesses, swellings, and tumors.

To make a compress, soak a cloth in a hot infusion or decoction, wring out the excess liquid, and apply the cloth to the area. Replace the compress when it cools by dipping again into the hot infusion or decoction. As with a poultice, a hot-water bottle placed over the preparation helps retain the heat.

**Washes** are just what they sound like: you wash the area with an infusion or decoction. For example, you might want to use an eyewash for conjunctivitis or a wash for a skin infection such as ringworm. Washes are an effective and simple external remedy.

### Alcohol Bases

Alcohol is used for making tinctures, which are concentrated alcohol extracts of herbs. It is a valuable menstruum because certain plant substances can be extracted only by alcohol.

Tinctures are concentrated, quick acting, and convenient (they can easily be transported in a small bottle), and they have a shelf life of many years. Because they are so concentrated, only a few drops are needed, making them particularly convenient for those who can't easily prepare infusions or decoctions. They are not, however, used when the nutritional aspects of herbs are being sought. For this, one should use teas, infusions, decoctions, and syrups.

The amount of alcohol ingested when taking tinctures is fairly insignificant, but if you are concerned, many tinctures can now be purchased in a glycerin base, which has no alcohol and a slightly sweet taste.

Making tinctures at home is fun and much less expensive than buying them. Because tinctures made with fresh plant material are superior to those made from dried herbs, obtain fresh herbs for your homemade tinctures. The best alcohol to use is 100-proof vodka, which is 50 percent alcohol and 50 percent water. Grain alcohol (almost 200 proof) or brandy can also be used. Brandy is nice for use in tinctures that will be given to very young kids because it is sweet and mildly warming, and it lacks a sharp alcohol taste.

**Tinctures:** If you have gathered the herbs yourself, clean them by picking out damaged parts and brushing dirt off roots. Do not wash above-ground plant parts. Roots, stems, and bark need to be chopped. Place about 2 ounces of plant material in a pint jar. Fill the jar to the top with alcohol to lessen the possibility of spoilage. Cap the jar tightly and label it with the name of the herb, alcohol content, and the date. Store it where it won't be exposed to direct sunlight, and give it a gentle shake every few days. If you see the liquid level going down, top off the jar with some more alcohol.

The moon exerts ongoing effects on the Earth, including the level of oceans and the growth of plants, as well as our own internal regulatory mechanisms and our hormones. It is also said to influence tincture making. It may therefore be beneficial to honor the effects of the moon by allowing our tinctures to rest for at least one complete moon cycle before using, going from one new moon to the next, or preferably for a full six weeks, from one new moon to the full moon six weeks later.

After two to six weeks, strain the alcohol tincture from the plant material. This usually requires some vigorous wringing of the herbs in cheesecloth or cotton muslin to extract as much of the liquid as possible. Pour your tincture into well-labeled glass jars or tincture bottles (the jars need not be filled to the top) and store in a cool, dark place such as a pantry or the refrigerator.

Dosage of a tincture depends on the herbs used, the condition being treated, and the person's age and weight. Usually a dose between 5 and 25 drops is taken four times a day. Tinctures remain good for a minimum of two to three years.

> CAUTION: Store your tinctures out of reach of children as an overdose might make them sick.

**Liniments:** These are tinctures prepared for external use in the treatment of muscle and ligament trauma. They tend to contain herbs that act as local stimulants (for example, angelica, cinnamon, wintergreen, cayenne, and calendula) in order to bring deep warmth to the affected area and disperse blood congestion to reduce bruising. The alcohol (use vodka or another 100-proof alcohol) makes them quick absorbing and penetrating. Prepare as for tinctures, or add essential oils to an alcohol base. Apply by rubbing enough into the skin to cover the sore or bruised area. Do not use on broken skin.

### Oil Bases

Herbal oils, salves, and ointments can be made at home. Essential oils are highly concentrated plant extracts that cannot easily be made at home and are rarely used internally because their strength can be fatal. I have occasionally suggested the use of essential oils in this book as external remedies, and caution you to store them out of the reach of children.

**Herbal oils** are vegetable oils in which herbs have been infused. They are different from essential oils, which are derived by extracting large volumes of concentrated, active chemical ingredients from plants. Herbal oils are used in the treatment of sore muscles, sprains, aches, infections, and irritated skin, as well as for massage. Many herbal oils mentioned in this book can be used on broken skin, although arnica oil cannot.

To make an herbal oil, fill a clean and totally dry jar with dry herbs. Now fill the jar to the brim with oil. Almond, olive, and sesame oils are the most commonly used, but any vegetable oil is acceptable. Store at room temperature in partial sunlight for one to four weeks. Some herbs, such as garlic and rosemary, will keep well in oil for the longer time span, while other herbs, particularly the more delicate plants and plant parts such as chickweed and rose petals, will begin to spoil after a week. Hot weather will cause the plants and oil to spoil more quickly, whereas plants extracted in a cool environment will keep longer before you decant them. Direct light and heat should be avoided. Infuse and store on a surface that will not be damaged by any oil seepage that may occur. At the end of the given time period, strain well and store in a cool, dark place or refrigerate. Oils will keep for up to a year or more and are considered good as long as they have not turned rancid. A rancid oil has a peculiar smell that is distinctly different from either the smell of the fresh oil or the plant being steeped. If you suspect that your oil has turned, discard it and begin anew.

**Salves** are used for healing skin injuries: wounds, burns, stings, rashes, sores, and the like. Salve can be made a few different ways, all of which are effective. This first method is preferable because it requires less time than the others and thus retains more of the subtle properties of the herbs. Prepare an herbal oil from your desired ingredients and pour it into a small pot. To this add grated beeswax, 1 tablespoon per ounce of oil. Heat over a low flame until the wax is melted. To test for readiness, put a small amount onto a teaspoon and place it in the refrigerator. After a minute, it will harden to its finished consistency. Salve should be firm and solid but not so hard that it won't melt into your skin. If the consistency is correct, pour your salve into small jars, cool to room temperature, cover, and store. If your salve is too soft, add more beeswax; if it is too hard, add more oil. Avoid overheating your beeswax.

A second method is to place about an ounce of herbs and $^1/_3$ cup of oil in a small pot. Simmer for two hours on a very low flame with the pot covered. Add a bit of oil if necessary, and watch carefully to avoid scorching. After cooking, strain the herbs well through a cotton cloth or cheesecloth, squeezing as much of the oil as possible out of the plant material. You may need to let the oil cool before this can be done. Clean the pot and dry it (discarding the used plant material) and then pour the oil back in, adding a couple tablespoons of grated beeswax. Melt this over a low flame, stirring constantly. Check for readiness as in the first method and then bottle and store.

Another method requires less watching. Mix 4 ounces of oil, 1 ounce of herbs, and $^1/_2$ ounce of beeswax in an ovenproof pot. Cover the pot and bake the mixture for about three hours at 250°F. Strain through cheesecloth, bottle, and store.

Salves will keep for a couple of years if stored in the refrigerator, about a year if not. To extend the life of your salve to the full two years, you can add 1 teaspoon of vitamin E oil or 1 to 2 tablespoons of an herbal tincture per 4 ounces of salve (while still warm, before bottling). Any herbal tincture will work, as it is the alcohol that helps preserve it, but to increase the healing qualities of your salve, use a tincture with either skin-healing or antimicrobial properties. Echinacea and calendula tinctures make good choices for use in herbal salves.

**Ointments** are prepared exactly like salves, but less beeswax is used in order to obtain a softer product. Cutting the amount of beeswax by half should yield a desirable consistency.

When you experiment in your kitchen pharmacy, above all enjoy yourself. Of course it is best not to be wasteful, but don't worry if you make a mistake and have to discard something. Compost piles are very forgiving. Try to be patient and learn from your mistakes. Be persistent; the rewards are worth it!

# Common and Latin Names for Herbs in This Book

$\ggg\!\!\!\!\lll$

*Many plants may have the same common name,* and any given plant may have a number of common names. A plant's Latin name (also known as the *botanical* or *horticultural* name) is its internationally recognized name. When purchasing herbs, check their Latin names to ensure that you are using the correct plants in your herbal preparations.

Alfalfa: *Medicago sativa*

Anise: *Pimpinella anisum*

Astragalus: *Astragalus membranaceus*

Bayberry: *Myrica cerifera*

Beth root: *Trillium* spp.

Black cohosh: *Actaea racemusa, syn. Cimicifuga racemosa*

Black haw: *Viburnum prunifolium*

Black walnut: *Juglans nigra*

Blessed thistle: *Cnicus benedictus*

Blue cohosh: *Caulophyllum thalictroides*

Borage: *Borago officinalis*

Bupleurum: *Bupleurum falcatum*

Burdock: *Arctium lappa*

Calendula: *Calendula officinalis*

Catnip: *Nepeta cataria*

Chamomile: *Anthemis nobilis; Matricaria chamomilla*

Chasteberry: *Vitex agnus-castus*

Chickweed: *Stellaria media*

Cinnamon: *Cinnamomum zeylanicum*

Cleavers: *Galium aparine*

Comfrey: *Symphytum officinale*

Cramp bark: *Viburnum opulus*

Dandelion: *Taraxacum officinale*

Dong quai: *Angelica sinensis*

Echinacea: *Echinacea angustifolia*

Elder: *Sambucus nigra*

False unicorn: *Chamaelirium luteum*

Fennel: *Foeniculum vulgare*

Fenugreek: *Trigonella foenum-graecum*

Flaxseed: *Linum usitatissimum*

Gentian: *Gentian officinalis*

Ginger: *Zingiber officinale*

Ginseng: *Panax quinquefolium*

Goldenseal: *Hydrastis canadensis*

Hawthorn: *Crataegus oxyacantha*

Hops: *Humulus lupulus*

Irish moss: *Chondrus crispus*

Kudzu: *Pueraria lobata*

Lady's mantle: *Alchemilla vulgaris*

Lady's slipper: *Cypripedium pubescens*

Lavender: *Lavandula officinalis*

Lemon balm: *Melissa officinalis*

Lemon grass: *Cymbopogon citratus*

Licorice: *Glycyrrhiza glabra*

Liferoot: *Senecio aureus*

Lime (linden) blossom: *Tiliax europaea*

Lobelia: *Lobelia inflata*

Marshmallow: *Althaea officinalis*

Meadowsweet: *Filipendula ulmaria*

Motherwort: *Leonurus cardiaca*

Myrrh: *Commiphora molmol*

Nettle: *Urtica dioica*

Oatstraw: *Avena sativa*

Parsley: *Petroselinum crispum*

Partridge berry: *Mitchella repens*

Passionflower: *Passiflora incarnata*

Peony: *Paeonia* spp.

Peppermint: *Menthax piperita*

Plantain: *Plantago major*

Red clover: *Trifolium pratense*

Red raspberry: *Rubus idaeus*

Rehmannia: *Rehmannia glutinosa*

Rose: *Rosa canina*

Rosemary: *Rosmarinus officinalis*

Sage: *Salvia officinalis*

Sarsaparilla: *Smilax officinalis*

Saw palmetto: *Serenoa serrulata*

Shepherd's purse: *Capsella bursa-pastoris*

Skullcap: *Scutellaria laterifolia*

Slippery elm: *Ulmus fulva*

Spearmint: *Mentha spicata*

Spikenard: *Aralia racemosa*

St. John's wort: *Hypericum perforatum*

Thyme: *Thymus vulgaris*

Usnea: *Usnea barbata*

Uva ursi: *Arctostaphylos uva-ursi*

Valerian: *Valeriana officinalis*

Vervain: *Verbena officinalis*

White oak: *Quercus alba*

Wild yam: *Dioscorea villosa*

Witch hazel: *Hamamelis virginiana*

Wood betony: *Betonica officinalis*

Yarrow: *Achillea millefolium*

Yellow dock: *Rumex crispus*

# Resources

The *following organizations* and companies provide high-quality services and are reputable resources in the midwifery and herbal communities. Inclusion here, however, does not necessarily imply endorsement all of the opinions, products, or services provided by these companies, and is not a direct referral to any individual practitioners.

## CHILDBIRTH EDUCATION AND DOULA ORGANIZATIONS

### Birth Arts International

www.birtharts.com/index.htm
demetria@birtharts.com
(866) 300-4372
Demetria Clark, BAI
501 Lindsey St.
Reidsville, NC 27320

### Bradley Method of Husband-Coached Childbirth

www.bradleybirth.com
(818) 788-6662; 800-4-A-BIRTH
P.O. Box 5224
Sherman Oaks, CA 91413-5224

### CAPPA

www.cappa.net
info@cappa.net
(770) 932-7281
P.O. Box 2406
Buford, GA 30515

### International Childbirth Education Association (ICEA)

www.icea.org
info@icea.org
(919) 863-9487; (800) 624-4934
500 Sunday Dr., Suite 102
Raleigh, NC 27607

### Lamaze

www.lamazeinternational.org/ContactUs
info@lamaze.org
(202) 367-1128; (800) 368-4404
2025 M St., NW, Suite 800
Washington, DC 20036-3309

## HERBAL ORGANIZATIONS

### American Botanical Council
http://abc.herbalgram.org/site/PageServer
abc@herbalgram.org
(512) 926-4900
6200 Manor Rd,
Austin, TX 78723

### American Herbalists Guild (AHG)
www.americanherbalistsguild.com
office@americanherbalistsguild.com
(617) 520-4372
14 Waverly Ct.
Asheville, NC 28805

### United Plant Savers
www.unitedplantsavers.org
office@UnitedPlantSavers.org
(802) 476-6467
P.O. Box 400
East Barre, VT 05649

## HERBAL PRODUCT RESOURCES

### Frontier Natural Products Co-op
www.frontiercoop.com
customercare@frontiercoop.com
(800) 669-3275
P.O. Box 299
3021 78th St.
Norway, IA 52318

### Herbalists & Alchemists
www.herbalist-alchemist.com
herbalist@nac.net
(908) 689-9020
51 South Wandling Ave.
Washington, NJ 07882

### Herb Pharm
www.herb-pharm.com
info@herb-pharm.com
(541) 846-6262
orders: (800) 348-4372
P.O. Box 116
Williams, OR 97544

### Maine Seaweed
www.theseaweedman.com
hanson.larch@gmail.com
(207) 546-2875
P.O. Box 57
Steuben, ME 04680

### Motherlove
www.motherlove.com
mother@motherlove.com
(970) 493-2892
3101 Kintzley Ct., Suite S
P.O. Box 101
Laporte, CO 80535

### Mountain Rose Herbs
www.mountainroseherbs.com
customerservice@mountainroseherbs.com
(800) 879-3337
international: (541) 741-7307
P.O. Box 50220
Eugene, OR 97405

## HYPNOBIRTHING

### Birthing From Within
www.birthingfromwithin.com
contact@birthingfromwithin.com
(805) 964-6611
P.O. Box 60259
Santa Barbara, CA 93160

**HypnoBirthing Institute**

www.hypnobirthing.com

hypnobirthing@hypnobirthing.com

(603) 856-8792; (603) 856-8341

office hours: 8:00am–3:00pm

110-2 Sheep Davis Rd.

Pembroke, NH 03275

**International Center for Traditional Childbearing (ICTC)**

www.blackmidwives.org

ictc@ictcmidwives.org

(503) 460-9324

P.O. Box 11923

Portland, OR 97211

## MAGAZINES

*Birthnbabies*

http://store.birthnbabies.com/
  subscription

*Compleat Mother*

www.compleatmother.com

*The Herb Quarterly*

www.herbquarterly.com

*Herbs for Health*

www.herbsforhealth.com

*Journal of the American Herbalist Guild*

www.americanherbalistsguild.com

*Midwifery Today*

www.midwiferytoday.com

*Natural Mother Magazine*

www.naturalmothermagazine.com

*Sacred Pregnancy*

www.sacredpregnancy.com

*Squat*

http://squatbirthjournal.org

## MIDWIFERY ORGANIZATIONS

**Citizens for Midwifery**

http://cfmidwifery.org/index.aspx

info@cfmidwifery.org

(888) 236-4880

P.O. Box 82227

Athens, GA 30608-2227

**Midwives Alliance of North America (MANA)**

www.mana.org

info@mana.org

(888) 923-MANA [(888) 923-6262]

1500 Sunday Dr., Suite 102

Raleigh, NC 27607

**North American Registry of Midwives (NARM)**

http://narm.org

info@narm.org

(888) 842-4784; (770) 381-9051

5257 Rosestone Dr.

Lilburn, GA 30047

**Postpartum Support International**

www.postpartum.net

support and resources:
  support@postpartum.net

(503) 894-9453

support helpline: (800) 944-4773

6706 SW 54th Ave.

Portland, OR 97219

## PREGNANCY AND BIRTH SUPPLIES FOR MIDWIVES AND HOME-BIRTH MAMAS

### BirthwithLove Midwifery Supplies

www.birthwithlove.com

orders@birthwithlove.com

(800) 434-4915

### Cascade HealthCare Products

www.1cascade.com

customerserviceatcascade@gmail.com

(503) 595-1720

1826 NW 18th Ave,

Portland, OR 97209

### Everything Birth

www.everythingbirth.com/
   Home-Birth-Kits.html

info@everythingbirth.com

(800) 370-1683

international calls must use
   (207) 781-2115

P.O. Box 66781

Falmouth, ME 04105

### Mama Goddess Birth Shop

www.mamagoddessbirthshop.com

info@mamagoddess.com

(888) 588-7417

## PREGNANCY AND BIRTH WEBSITES AND BLOGS

### About.com Pregnancy

http://pregnancy.about.com

### American Baby Magazine

www.parents.com/
   american-baby-magazine

### Association for Pre- & Perinatal Psychology and Health (APPPAH)

http://birthpsychology.com

consultant@birthpsychology.com

P.O. Box 1398

Forestville, CA 95436

### BabyCenter

www.babycenter.com

### BellyBelly.com

www.bellybelly.com.au

### Birth Without Fear—Empowering Women to Make Informed Choices

http://birthwithoutfearblog.com

### Birthing the Future

http://birthingthefuture.org

Suzanne Arms, Founder–Director

suzannebirthing@gmail.com

(970) 884-4005

P.O. Box 1040

Bayfield, CO 81122

### The Bump

www.thebump.com

### Childbirth Connection

www.childbirthconnection.org

### Coalition for Improving Maternity Services (CIMS)

www.motherfriendly.org

### Evidence-Based Birth

http://evidencebasedbirth.com/home

**International Cesarean Awareness Network (ICAN)**
www.ican-online.org
(800) 686-ICAN [(800) 686-4226]
P.O. Box 31423
St. Louis, MO 63131

**La Leche League International**
www.lalecheleague.org
(847) 519-7730; (800) LALECHE
[(800) 525-3243]
957 N. Plum Grove Rd.
Schaumburg, IL 60173

**Lamaze**
www.lamaze.org

**Midwife Thinking**
http://midwifethinking.com

**Midwifery Today**
www.midwiferytoday.com

**Peggy O'Mara**
www.peggyomara.com

**Science & Sensibility**
www.scienceandsensibility.org

**Waterbirth International**
www.waterbirth.org
(954) 821-9125
P.O. Box 5578
Lighthouse Point, FL 33074

**What to Expect**
www.whattoexpect.com/what-to-expect/
    landing-page.aspx

## WOMEN'S HERBAL EDUCATION

**Herbal Medicine for Women**
http://herbalmedicineforwomen.com

# Bibliography

Achterberg, Jeanne. 1991. *Woman as Healer*. Boston: Shambhala Publications.

Allaire, Alexander D. 2001. Complementary and alternative medicine in the labor and delivery suite. *Clinical Obstetrics and Gynecology* 44(4)(Dec):681–91.

Allaire, Alexander D., Merry-K Moos, Steven R. Wells. 2000. Complementary and alternative medicine in pregnancy: A survey of North Carolina certified nurse-midwives. *Obstetrics & Gynecology* 95(1)(Jan):19–23.

Arms, Suzanne. 1975. *Immaculate Deception*. New York: Bantam Books.

_____. 1994. *Immaculate Deception II: A Fresh Look at Childbirth*. Berkeley, CA: Celestial Arts.

Backon, J. 1991. Ginger in preventing nausea and vomiting of pregnancy: A caveat due to its thromboxane synthetase activity and effect on testosterone binding. *European Journal of Obstetrics and Gynecology and Reproductive Biology* 42(Nov):54, 163–64.

Baker, Jeannine P. 1991. *Deep Ecology of Childbirth*. Monroe, UT: Freestone Publishing, 1991.

_____. 1979. *Hygieia: A Woman's Herbal*. Monroe, UT: Freestone Publishing.

_____. 1986. *Prenatal Yoga and Natural Childbirth*. Berkeley, CA: North Atlantic.

Baker, Jeannine P., F. Baker, and T. Slayton. 1986. *Conscious Conception*. Sevier, UT: Freestone Publishing.

Baker, Jeannine Parvati and Frederick Baker. *Conscious Conception: Elemental Journey through the Labyrinth of Sexuality*. Monroe, UT: Freestone Pub. Co., 1986.

Balacs, Tony. 1992. Safety in pregnancy. *International Journal of Aromatherapy* 4(1)(Spring):12–15.

Baldwin, Rahima. 1986. *Special Delivery*. Berkeley, CA: Celestial Arts.

Baldwin, Rahima, and Terra Palmarini. 1986. *Pregnant Feelings*. Berkeley, CA: Celestial Arts.

Ballantine, Rudolph. 1978. *Diet and Nutrition*. Honesdale, PA: Himalaya International Institute.

Bates, Barbara. 1983. *A Guide to the Physical Examination*. 3d ed. Philadelphia: J. B. Lippincott Co.

Beinfield, Harriet, and E. Korngold. 1991. B*etween Heaven and Earth: A Guide to Chinese Medicine*. New York: Ballantine Books.

Bennett, Jennifer. 1991. *Lilies of the Hearth*. Willowdale, Ontario, Canada: Camden House Publishing.

Bing, Elizabeth, and Libby Colman. 1977. *Making Love During Pregnancy*. New York: Bantam Books.

Blumburg, Stephen J., Susanna N. Visser, Melissa L. Danielson, Rebecca H. Bitsko, Joseph R. Holbrook, Michael D. Kogan, Reem M. Ghandour, and Ruth Perou. "Trends in the Parent-Report of Health Care Provider-Diagnosed and Medicated Attention-Deficit/Hyperactivity Disorder: United States, 2003–2011." *Journal of the American Academy of Child & Adolescent Psychiatry*, 53, no. 1 (January 2014): 34-46.e2.

Boston Women's Health Book Collective. 1998. *Our Bodies, Ourselves for the New Century*. New York: Simon & Schuster.

Boston Women's Health Collective and Judy Norsigian. *Our Bodies, Ourselves*. New York: Touchstone, 2011.

Brewer, Gail S., and Tom Brewer. 1977. *What Every Pregnant Woman Should Know: The Truth about Diet and Drugs in Pregnancy*. New York: Penguin Books.

Brinker, Francis. 1998. *Herb Contraindications and Drug Interactions*. 2d ed. Sandy, OR: Eclectic Medical Publications.

Brooke, Elizabeth. 1992. *Herbal Therapy for Women*. London, England: Thorsons.

Buckley, Kathleen, and Nancy W. Kulb. 1983. *Handbook of Maternal Newborn Nursing*. New York: John Wiley and Sons.

Cardini, Francesco, and Huang Weixin. 1998. Moxibustion for correction of breech presentation: A randomized control trial. *Journal of the American Medical Association* 280(18)(Nov 11):1580–84.

Carlsson, Christopher P., et al. 2000. Manual acupuncture reduces hyperemesis gravidarum: A placebo-controlled, randomized, single-blind, crossover study. *Journal of Pain Symptom Management* 20(4)(Oct):273–79.

Cavanagh, Dennis, Ralph Woods, Timothy O'Connor, and Robert Knuppel. 1982. *Obstetric Emergencies*. Philadelphia: Harper and Row.

CDC. "Prevalence of Autism Spectrum Disorder Among Children Aged 8 Years—Autism and Developmental Disabilities Monitoring Network." *MMWR* 2014; 63 (No. SS 2): 1-21.

Cohen, Nancy W. *Open Season*. 1991. New York: Greenwood, Bergin, and Garvey.

Cohen, Nancy W., and Lois Estner. 1983. *Silent Knife*. New York: Greenwood, Bergin, and Garvey.

Corda, Murshida. 1987. *Cradle of Heaven: Psychological and Spiritual Dimensions of Conception, Pregnancy, and Birth*. Lebanon Springs, NY: Omega.

Dabelea, Dana, Elizabeth J. Mayer-Davis, Sharon Saydah, Giuseppina Imperatore, Barbara Linder, Jasmin Divers, Ronny Bell, Angela Badaru, Jennifer W. Talton, Tessa Crume, Angela D. Liese, Anwar T. Merchant, Jean M. Lawrence, Kristi Reynolds, Lawrence

Dolan, Lenna L. Liu, and Richard F. Hamman. "Prevalence of Type 1 and Type 2 Diabetes Among Children and Adolescents From 2001 to 2009." JAMA, 2014;311(17):1778-1786. doi:10.1001/jama.2014.3201.

Dale, Alisa, and Sheila Cornwell. 1994. The role of lavender oil in relieving perineal discomfort following childbirth: A blind randomized clinical trial. *Journal of Advanced Nursing* 19(1)(Jan):89–96.

Davis, Elizabeth. 1987. *Heart and Hands: A Midwife's Guide to Pregnancy and Birth*. Berkeley, CA: Celestial Arts.

Davis, Elizabeth. *Heart and Hands: A Midwife's Guide to Pregnancy and Birth*. Berkeley: Celestial Arts, 2004.

_____. 1989. *Women's Intuition*. Berkeley, CA: Celestial Arts.

Davis-Floyd, Robbie. 1992. *Birth as an American Right of Passage*. Berkeley, CA: University of California Press.

Dharmananda, Subhuti. 1989. *Treatment of Infertility and Miscarriage with Chinese Herbs*. Portland, OR: Institute for Traditional Medicine and Preventive Health Care.

_____. 1986. *Your Nature, Your Health: Chinese Herbs in Constitutional Therapy*. Portland, OR: Institute for Traditional Medicine and Preventive Health Care.

Dick-Read, Grantly. 1979. *Childbirth Without Fear*. New York: Harper and Row.

Dunham, Carroll. 1991. *Mamatoto: A Celebration of Birth*. New York: Penguin USA, Viking.

Ehrenreich, Barbara, and Deidre English. 1973. *Witches, Midwives, and Nurses: A History of Women Healers*. New York: Feminist Press at the City University of New York.

Eisenberg, Arlene, H. E. Murkoff, and S. E. Hathaway. 1986. *What to Eat When You're Expecting*. New York: Workman Publishing.

Eisler, Riane. *The Chalice and the Blade: Our History, Our Future*. Cambridge, MA: Harper & Row, 1988.

Ellingwood, Finley. 1998. *American Materia Medica, Therapeutics and Pharmacognosy*, 11th ed. Reprint. Sandy, OR: Eclectic Medical Publications.

Federation of Feminist Women's Health Centers. 1981. *A New View of a Woman's Body*. New York: Touchstone.

Felter, H. 1994. *The Eclectic Materia Medica, Pharmacology and Therapeutics*. 1922. Reprint. Sandy, OR: Eclectic Medical Publications.

Field, Tiffany, et al. 1977. Labor pain is reduced by massage therapy. *Journal of Psychosomatic Obstetrics and Gynecology* 18(4)(Dec):286–91.

Field, Tiffany, et al. 1999. Pregnant women benefit from massage therapy. *Journal of Psychosomatic Obstetrics and Gynecology* 20(1)(Mar):31–38.

Fischer-Rasmussen, W., S. K. Kjaer, C. Dahl, and U. Asping. 1991. Ginger treatment of hyperemesis gravidarum. *European Journal of Obstetrics, Gynecology, and Reproductive Biology* 38(Jan):19–24.

Flaws, Bob. 1986. *Free and Easy: Traditional Chinese Gynecology for American Women*. Boulder, CO: Blue Poppy Press.

_____. 1987. *A Handbook of Traditional Chinese Gynecology*. Boulder, CO: Blue Poppy Press.

_____. 1993. *The Path of Pregnancy*. Boulder, CO: Blue Poppy Press.

Foster, Steven, and J. Duke. 1990. *Eastern/Central Medicinal Plants*. Boston: Houghton Mifflin Co.

Francia, Luisa. 1991. *Dragontime: Magic and Mystery of Menstruation*. Woodstock, NY: Ash Tree Publishing.

Frawley, David, and V. Lad. 1986. *The Yoga of Herbs*. Santa Fe, NM: Lotus Light, Lotus Press.

Frye, Anne. 1995. *Care During Pregnancy*, vol. 1, *in Holistic Midwifery: A Comprehensive Textbook for Midwives in Homebirth Practice*. Portland, OR: Labrys Press.

_____. 1990. *Understanding Lab Work in the Childbearing Year*. New Haven, CT: Labrys Press.

Fulder, Stephen, and Meir Tenne. 1996. Ginger as an antinausea remedy in pregnancy: The issue of safety. *HerbalGram* 38(Fall):47–50.

Gallo, Michael, and Maumita Sarkar, et al. 2000. Pregnancy outcome following gestational exposure to echinacea. *Archives of Internal Medicine* 160(20)(13 Nov):3141–43.

Gallo, M., M. Sarkar, W. Au, K. Pietrzak, B. Comas, M. Smith, T.V. Jaeger, A. Einarson, and G. Koren. "Pregnancy Outcome Following Exposure to Echinacea: A Prospective Controlled Study." *Archives of Internal Medicine* 160, no. 20 (November 2000): 3141–3143.

Gardner, Zoë, and Michael McGuffin. *American Herbal Products Association's Botanical Safety Handbook*. Boca Raton, FL: CRC Press, 2013.

Gaskin, Ina May. 1980. *Spiritual Midwifery*. Summertown, TN: Book Publishing Co.

Gelis, Jacques. 1991. *History of Childbirth: Fertility, Pregnancy, and Birth in Early Modern Europe*. Boston: Northeastern University Press.

Gimbutas, Marija. *The Living Goddesses*. Edited by Miriam Robbins Dexter. Berkeley: University of California Press, 2001.

Gladstar, Rosemary. 1993. *Herbal Healing for Women*. New York: Simon and Schuster.

Goer, Henci. 1995. *Obstetric Myths versus Research Realities: A Guide to the Medical Literature*. Westport, CT: Greenwood, Bergin, and Garvey.

Goldsmith, Judith. 1984. *Childbirth Wisdom from the World's Oldest Societies*. New York: Congdon and Weed.

Grossinger, Richard. 1986. *Embryogenesis*. Berkeley, CA: North Atlantic Books.

Harrison, Michelle. 1982. *A Woman in Residence*. New York: Penguin.

Hazell, Lester. 1976. *Commonsense Childbirth*. New York: Berkley Books.

Hedegaard M. 1999. Life style, work and stress, and pregnancy outcome. *Current Opinion in Gynecology* 11(6)(Dec):553–56.

Ho, C.-M., S.-S. Hseu, S.-K. Tsai, T.-Y. Lee. 1996. Effect of P-6 acupressure on prevention of nausea and vomiting after epidural morphine for post–cesarean section pain relief. *Acta Anaesthesiologica Scandinavica* 40(3)(Mar):372–75.

Hobbs, Valerie. 1982. *Complications of Labor and Delivery*. Ann Arbor, MI: Informed Homebirth and Parenting.

———. 1981. *Herbs for Women: A Guide for Lay Midwives*. Ann Arbor, MI: Informed Homebirth and Parenting.

Hochstrasser, B., and P. Mattman. 1999. Mainstream medicine versus complementary medicine (homeopathic) intervention: A critical methodology study of pregnancy. *Forsch Komplementarmed* 6(6)(supplement 1, Feb):20–22.

Hoffman, David. 1983. *The Holistic Herbal*. Moray, Scotland: Findhorn Press.

Hollis, B.W., D. Johnson, T.C. Hulsey, M. Ebeling, and C.L. Wagner. "Vitamin D supplementation during pregnancy: double blind, randomized clinical trial of safety and effectiveness." J Bone Miner Res 26, no. 12 (Dec 2011): 2341-2357.

Huxley, Laura. 1992. *The Child of Your Dreams*. Rochester, VT: Inner Traditions, Destiny Books.

Jensen, Margaret D., Ralph Benson, and Irene Bobak. 1981. *Maternity Care: The Nurse and the Family*. St. Louis: Mosby.

Jewell, D., and G. Young. 1997. Interventions for Nausea and Vomiting in Early Pregnancy. In Jim P. Neilson, Caroline Crowther, Ellen Hodnett, Justus Hofmeyr, and M. Keirse, eds. *Pregnancy and Childbirth Module of the Cochrane Database of Systematic Reviews, The Cochrane Collaboration*, issue 2. Oxford, England: Update Software.

Katz-Rothman, Barbara. 1993. *The Encyclopedia of Childbearing*. New York: Henry Holt.

Keating, Angela, and Ronald Chez. 2002. Ginger syrup as an antiemetic in early pregnancy. *Alternative Therapies in Health and Medicine* 8(5)(Sep–Oct):89–91.

Kirschmann, John, and L. Dunne. 1984. *Nutrition Almanac*. New York: McGraw-Hill.

Kitzinger, Sheila. 1979. *Birth at Home*. New York: Penguin.

———. 1983. *The Complete Book of Pregnancy and Childbirth*. New York: Alfred A. Knopf.

———. 1979. *Education and Counseling for Childbirth*. New York: Schocken Books.

Klaus, Marshall, and John Kennell. 1983. *Bonding*. New York: Penguin USA, Plume.

Koehler, Nan. 1985. *Artemis Speaks: VBAC Stories and Natural Childbirth Information*. Occidental, CA: Jerald R. Brown.

Kushi, Michio, and Aveline Kushi. 1983. *Macrobiotic Pregnancy and Care of the Newborn*. New York: Japan Publishing.

La Leche League. 1981. *The Womanly Art of Breastfeeding*. New York: Plume.

Leboyer, Frederick. 1978. *Inner Beauty, Inner Light: Yoga for Pregnant Women*. New York: Alfred A. Knopf.

Liedloff, Jean. 1977. *The Continuum Concept*. Reading, MA: Addison-Wesley Publishing Co.

Litoff, J. B. 1986. *The American Midwife Debate*. New York: Greenwood Press.

Louden, Jennifer. 1994. *The Couple's Comfort Book*. San Francisco: HarperCollins.

———. 1992. *The Woman's Comfort Book*. New York: HarperCollins.

Low Dog, Tieraona. 2001. *An Integrative Approach to Women's Health*. Albuquerque, NM: Integrative Medical Education Associates.

Low Dog, T. *Women's Health in Complementary and Integrative Medicine: A Clinical Guide*. St. Louis, MO: Elsevier, 2004.

Madaras, Lynda, and Jane Patterson. 1984. *Womancare: A Gynecological Guide to Your Body*. New York: Avon Books.

Magee, Laura A., Paolo Mazzotta, and Gideon Koren. 2002. Evidence-based view of safety and effectiveness of pharmacologic therapy for nausea and vomiting of pregnancy (NVP). *American Journal of Obstetrics and Gynecology* 185(5) (supplement understanding, May):S256–61.

Mariechild, Diane. 1981. *MotherWit*. Trumansburg, NY: The Crossing Press.

McClure, Vimala Schneider. 1989. *Infant Massage*. New York: Bantam Books.

McGuffin, M., et al. 1997. *Botanical Safety Handbook*. New York: CRC Press.

McIntyre, Anne. 1992. *The Herbal for Mother and Child*. Rockport, MA: Element Books.

Meek, Leslie R., Kristi M. Burda, and Erin Paster. 2000. Effects of prenatal stress on development in mice: Maturation and learning. *Physiology & Behavior* 71(5) (Dec):543–49.

Meltzer, Donna I. 2000. Complementary therapies for nausea and vomiting in early pregnancy. *Family Practice* 17(6)(Dec):570–73.

Mendelsohn, Robert. 1984. *How to Raise a Healthy Child in Spite of Your Doctor*. New York: Ballantine Books.

_____. 1982. *MalePractice: How Doctors Manipulate Women*. Chicago: Contemporary Books.

Merchant, Carolyn. 1980. *The Death of Nature: Women, Ecology, and the Scientific Revolution*. San Francisco: HarperSanFrancisco.

Miller, Jonathan, and D. Pelham. 1984. *The Facts of Life*. New York: Penguin USA, Viking.

Mills, S., and K. Bone. 2000. *Principles and Practice of Phytotherapy: Modern Herbal Medicine*. Edinburgh, Scotland: Churchill Livingstone.

Mitford, Jessica. 1992. *The American Way of Birth*. New York: Dutton/Signet.

Montagu, Ashley. 1981. *Growing Young*. New York: McGraw-Hill.

Moskowitz, Richard. 1992. *Homeopathic Medicines for Pregnancy and Childbirth*. Berkeley: North Atlantic Press.

Murphy, Patricia Aikens. 1998. Alternative therapies for nausea and vomiting of pregnancy. *Obstetrics & Gynecology* 91(1)(Jan):149–55.

National Research Council and Institute of Medicine. *U.S. Health in International Perspective: Shorter Lives, Poorer Health*. Washington, DC: The National Academies Press, 2013.

Niebyl, Jennifer R., and T. Murphy Goodwin. 2002. Overview of nausea and vomiting of pregnancy with an emphasis on vitamins. *American Journal of Obstetrics and Gynecology* 186(5) (supplement understanding, May):S253–55.

Nissim, Rina. 1986. *Natural Healing in Gynecology.* New York: Pandora Press.

Noble, Elizabeth. 1983. *Childbirth with Insight.* Boston: Houghton Mifflin Co.

_____. 1982. *Essential Exercises for the Childbearing Year.* Boston: Houghton Mifflin Co.

Noble, Vicki. 1991. *Shakti Woman.* San Francisco: HarperSanFrancisco.

_____. 1993. *Uncoiling the Snake.* San Francisco: HarperCollins.

Noble, Vicki. *Shakti Woman: Feeling Our Fire, Healing Our World – The New Female Shamanism.* San Francisco: HarperSanFrancisco, 1991.

Nofziger, Margaret. 1979. *A Cooperative Method of Natural Birth Control.* Summertown, TN: Book Publishing Co.

_____. 1982. *The Fertility Question.* Summertown, TN: Book Publishing Co.

Norheim, Arne Johan, Erik Jesman Pedersen, Vinjar Fonnebo, and Lillian Berge. 2001. Acupressure treatment of morning sickness in pregnancy: A randomised, double-blind, placebo-controlled study. *Scandinavian Journal of Primary Health Care* 19(1)(Mar):43–47.

Northrup, Christiane. 1998. *Women's Bodies, Women's Wisdom.* New York: Bantam Doubleday Dell.

Olds, Sally, Marcia London, and Patricia Ladewig. 1984. *Maternal Newborn Nursing.* Menlo Park, CA: Addison-Wesley.

Packer-Tursman, Judy. 2002. Alternative therapy struggles to bridge East-West divide. *Washington Post* 10 Nov 2002. www.washingtonpost.com/wp-dyn/articles/A36744-2002Nov10.html.

Panuthos, Claudia. 1984. *Transformation Through Birth.* South Hadley, MA: Greenwood, Bergin, and Garvey.

Parsons, Myra, Michele Simpson, and Terri Ponton. "Raspberry Leaf and Its Effect on Labour: Safety and Efficacy." *Australian College of Midwives Journal* 12, no. 3 (September 1999): 20–25.

Peterson, Gayle. 1984. *Birthing Normally.* Berkeley, CA: Mindbody Press.

Peterson, Gayle, and Lewis Mehl. 1984. *Pregnancy as Healing.* 2 vols. Berkeley, CA: Mindbody Press.

Price, Shirley. 1998. Using essential oils in professional practice. *Complementary Therapies in Nurse Midwifery* 4(5)(Oct):144–47.

Pritchard, Jack, and Paul MacDonald. 1976. *William's Obstetrics.* New York: Appleton-Century Croft.

Reeder, Sharon, Luigi Mastroianni Jr., and Leonide Martin. 1983. *Maternity Nursing.* Philadelphia: J. B. Lippincott Co.

Regutti, Amy. 2002. Pregnancy support with acupuncture and traditional Chinese medicine. *Infused: The Community Pharmacy Newsletter* 4(3)(Jun):1–3.

Rich, Adrienne. 1986. *Of Woman Born: Motherhood as Experience and Institution.* New York: W. W. Norton & Co.

Romm, Aviva. 1994. Healing a Uterine Prolapse. *The Birth Gazette* 10(3)(Summer):19–21.

_____. 2010. *Botanical Medicine for Women's Health*. St. Louis, Mo.: Churchill Livingstone/Elsevier.

_____. 2002. *Natural Health After Birth*. Rochester, VT: Healing Arts Press.

_____. 2003. *Naturally Healthy Babies and Children*. Berkeley, CA: Celestial Arts.

_____. 1998. *A Pocket Guide to Midwifery Care*. Freedom, CA: The Crossing Press.

_____. 2001. Treatment of incomplete miscarriage with botanical therapies and continuing reproductive care. *Journal of the American Herbalists Guild* 2(2)(Fall/Winter):16–17.

Romm, Aviva, and Jonathan Treasure. 2001. American Herbalists Guild professional member botanical therapeutics survey: Vitex agnus-castus. *Journal of the American Herbalists Guild* 2(2)(Fall/Winter):27–31.

Roscoe, Joseph A., and Sara E. Matteson. 2002. Acupressure and acustimulation bands for control of nausea review. *American Journal of Obstetrics and Gynecology* 185(5) (supplement understanding, May):S244–47.

Schwartz, Leni. 1991. *Bonding Before Birth*. Boston: Sigo Press.

Sears, William, and Martha Sears. 1994. *The Birth Book*. Boston: Little, Brown and Co.

Shuttle, Penelope, and P. Redgrove. 1986. *The Wise Wound*. New York: Grove Press.

Simpson, M., M. Parson, J. Greenwood, and K. Wade. "Raspberry Leaf in Pregnancy: Its Safety and Efficacy in Labor." *Journal of Midwifery & Women's Health* 46, no. 2 (March–April 2001): 51–59.

Slotnick, R. Nathan. 2001. Safe, successful nausea suppression in early pregnancy with P-6 acustimulation. *Journal of Reproductive Medicine* 46(9)(Sep):811–14.

Smith, C. A. 2001. Homoeopathy for Induction of Labour. Cochrane Database Syst Rev 4: CD00339.

Starhawk. *The Spiral Dance: A Rebirth of the Ancient Religion of the Goddess: 20th Anniversary Edition*. San Francisco: HarperSanFrancisco: 1999.

Stern, Robert M., Michael D. Jokerst, Eric R. Muth, and Chris Hollis. 2001. Acupressure relieves the symptoms of motion sickness and abnormal gastric activity. *Alternative Therapies in Health and Medicine* 7(4)(Jul–Aug):91–94.

Stillerman, Elaine. 1992. *Mother Massage*. New York: Dell Publishing.

Stone, Merlin. *When God Was a Woman*. New York: Harcourt Brace Jovanovich, 1978

Strong, Thomas H. 2001. Alternative therapies of morning sickness. *Clinical Obstetrics and Gynecology* 44(4)(Dec):653–60.

Stukane, Eileen. 1985. *The Dream Worlds of Pregnancy*. New York: Quill.

Taber, Ben-Zion. 1984. *Manual of Gynecologic and Obstetric Emergencies*. Philadelphia: W. B. Saunders Co.

Taylor, Dena. 1988. *Red Flower: Rethinking Menstruation*. Freedom, CA: The Crossing Press.

Thevenin, Tine. 1992. *The Family Bed: An Age-Old Concept in Child Rearing*. Garden City, NY: Avery.

Tierra, Lesley. 1992. *The Herbs of Life*. Freedom, CA: The Crossing Press.

Tierra, Michael. 1988. *Planetary Herbology*. Santa Fe, NM: Lotus Light Publications, Lotus Press.

_____. 1980. *The Way of Herbs*. Santa Cruz, CA: Orenda/Unity Press.

Tiran, D., and S. Mack. 1995. *Complementary Therapies for Pregnancy and Childbirth*. London, England: Bailliere Tindall.

Tortora, Gerard, and Nicholas Anagnostakos. 1984. *Principles of Anatomy and Physiology*. New York: Harper and Row.

Tyler, Varro. 1999. *Herbs of Choice: The Therapeutic Use of Phytomedicinals*. Binghamton, NY: Haworth Press.

Upton, Roy. 2001. Chaste Tree Fruit (*Vitex agnus-castus*). *American Herbal Pharmacopoeia and Therapeutic Compendium*. Santa Cruz, CA: American Herbal Pharmacopoeia.

_____. 2001. Cramp Bark (*Viburnum prunifolium*). *American Herbal Pharmacopoeia and Therapeutic Compendium*. Santa Cruz, CA: American Herbal Pharmacopoeia.

_____. 2002. Cranberry Fruit (*Vaccinium macrocarpon*). *American Herbal Pharmacopoeia and Therapeutic Compendium*. Santa Cruz, CA: American Herbal Pharmacopoeia.

Varney, Helen. 1980. *Nurse Midwifery*. Boston: Blackwell Scientific Publications.

Verny, Thomas, and John Kelly. 1981. *The Secret Life of the Unborn Child*. New York: Dell Publishing.

Vutyavanich, Teraporn, et al. 2001. Ginger for nausea and vomiting in pregnancy: Randomized, double-masked, placebo-controlled trial. *Obstetrics & Gynecology* 97(4)(Apr):577–82.

Vutyavanich, T., T. Kraisarin, and R. Ruangsri. "Ginger for Nausea and Vomiting in Pregnancy: Randomized, Doublemasked, Placebo-controlled Trial." *Obstetrics and Gynecology* 97, no. 4 (April 2001): 577–582.

Wagner, Marsden. 1994. *Pursuing the Birth Machine*. Camperdown, Australia: ACE Graphics.

Weed, Susun. 1989. *Healing Wise*. Woodstock, NY: Ash Tree Publishing.

_____. 1985. *Wise Woman Herbal for the Childbearing Year*. Woodstock, NY: Ash Tree Publishing.

Weiss, Rudolf. 1988. *Herbal Medicine*. Gothenburg, Sweden: AB Arcanum.

Werner, David. 1977. *Where There Is No Doctor: A Village Health Care Handbook*. Palo Alto, CA: Hesperian Foundation.

Wilkinson, Jenny M. 2000. What do we know about herbal morning sickness treatments? A literature survey. *Midwifery* 16(Sep):224–28.

Wilkinson, Susan, et al. 1999. An evaluation of aromatherapy massage in palliative care. *Palliative Medicine* 13(5)(Sep):409–17.

# About the Author

⫸⫷

AVIVA JILL ROMM, MD, is a physician and highly respected expert in botanical medicine, childbirth, women's health, and pediatrics. She practiced as a homebirth midwife and herbalist for more than twenty years, becoming one of the first certified professional midwives (CPM) in the United States. A graduate of Yale School of Medicine, where she received the Internal Medicine Award for "outstanding academic achievement and community service," Dr. Romm completed her intern year in Internal Medicine at Yale where she was instrumental in creating the school's first integrative medicine curriculum. Her numerous distinctions include serving as the President of the American Herbalists Guild for over a decade, serving as the Medical Director for American Herbal Pharmacopoeia (AHP), being on the advisory board for Yale Integrative Medicine, serving on the advisory board for the American Botanical Council, and teaching as an adjunct faculty for the Massachusetts College of Pharmacy.

# Index

Black haw
  for backache, 164
  for cramping, 167, 209
  for miscarriage prevention,
    213, 214
Bladder infections. *See* Urinary
    tract infections
Bleeding, vaginal
  in early pregnancy, 165–67, 178
  in late pregnancy, 168
  urinary tract infections
    and, 166
  *See also* Miscarriages
Blessed thistle, 84
Blessingway, 134–39
Blood root, 84
Blood sugar
  elevated, 186
  low (hypoglycemia), 72, 180,
    187, 188, 227
Blue cohosh, 84, 122, 218
BMI (Body Mass Index), 73
Body
  common beliefs and attitudes
    about, 11–12
  feelings and fears about, 15–16
  listening to your, 12–14
  and mind, relationship of,
    12–13
  moving joyously, 16–17
  physical changes in, 106–12
  preparing, for birth, 122–23
Body image
  importance of, 88–89
  media and, 11
  partners and, 142
  transforming negative to
    positive, 15, 17, 107
Body odor, 111
Boluses, 241–42
Bone loss, 112
Borage, 85
BPA (bisphenol A), 27, 54
Breastfeeding, preparing for,
    123–24
Breasts
  changes in, 106–7
  lumps in, 107
  sagging, 231
  sore, 106–7, 168–69
Breath, shortness of, 158, 159,
    178, 184
Breathing, deep, 102–3

Breech birth, 169–71, 180
Bridge pose, 93
Broom, 84
Buckthorn, 177
Burdock root, 64, 192–93
Butterfly pose, 92
Butternut, 84

## C

Caffeine
  calcium and, 167
  headaches and, 188
  iron and, 160
Calamus, 84
Calcium, 66, 70
  backaches and, 163
  caffeine and, 167
  cramping and, 167
  fats and, 60
  headaches and, 187, 188
  supplements, 188
Calendula, 84
  for herpes, 193
  after miscarriage, 221
  for vaginal infections, 241, 247
  for vaginal massage, 123
Calming Tea, 183
Cancer, 52
*Candida albicans*, 239
Caraway seeds, 68
Carbohydrates, 56, 58–59
Cardiovascular disease, 52
Cascara sagrada, 84
Castor oil, 177
Catnip
  for headaches, 189
  for herpes, 192
  for indigestion, 203
  for insomnia and anxiety,
    206, 221
  for leg cramps, 209
  as vitamin B$_1$ source, 62
Caul, 134
Cedar, 136
Centaur pose, 93
Cervix
  friable, 165
  polyps on, 165
Chamomile, 80
  as calcium source, 66
  Chamomile Tea, 205
  for cramping, 209
  for headaches, 189
  for herpes, 192

for high blood pressure, 198
  for indigestion, 203
  for insomnia and anxiety, 205,
    206, 219
  for muscle aches, 164
  for nausea, 229
  for relaxation, 182, 183, 221
  for vaginal massage, 123
Chasteberry, 213, 221
Cheese, 75
Chemical exposures, 25–27, 54
Chia-Lax, Morning, 177
Chickweed, 241
Chicory, 156
Childbirth. *See* Birth; Birthing
    practices
Childbirth education classes,
    49–50
Childbirth Providers of African
    Descent, 8
Chinese herbs, 85
Chlamydia, 237
Chlorophyll, liquid, 111, 161
Cholesterol, 60
Chorionic villi sampling (CVS),
    48–49
Cigarettes, 21
Cinnamon, 164, 186, 219
Cocoa butter, 231
Cohen, Nancy, 132
Cold foods, 212
Colds, 171–75
Cold sores. *See* Herpes
Colman, Libby, 143
Colostrum, 106
Coltsfoot, 84, 85, 202
Comfrey
  for herpes, 193
  as nutritional source, 61, 68
  for vaginal infections, 241
  warning about, 84, 85, 202
Complications, fears about, 181
Compresses, 258
Conception, 20, 22
Constipation, 158, 159, 175–77
  backaches and, 162, 163
  cramping and, 166
  headaches and, 187, 188
  recommendations for, 176–77
Contractions
  labor, 183
  normally occurring,
    110–11, 234

Fish, 26, 69, 75
Flu, 171–75
Folic acid, 63–64, 156–57
Food
  to avoid, 75
  cold, 212
  cravings, 14, 72
  guidelines for, 55–57
  hidden dangers in, 54–55
  journals, 74
  organic, 26
  *See also* Diets; Hunger;
    Nutrition
Foot baths, 258
Forward bends, 93
Fundus, 110

## G

Garlic
  for colds and viruses, 174
  Garlic Lemonade, 175
  Garlic-Onion-Ginger-Kudzu
    Tea, 175
  for high blood pressure, 196
  oil, 196
  for vaginal infections,
    240–41, 246
Gas, 166, 201
Gaskin, Ina May, 8
Gestational diabetes, 186
Ginger, 80
  effects of, 174
  Garlic-Onion-Ginger-Kudzu
    Tea, 175
  Ginger Tea, 175
  for nausea, 228–29
  warning about, 174
Ginseng, 84, 221
Glucose testing, 186
Goat's rue, 84
Goldenseal, 84, 242, 247
Gomasio, 195
Gonorrhea, 237
Gotu kola, 84
Ground ivy, 220
Group B strep, 242–49
Growth, personal, 128
Guilt, 182

## H

Hair, changes in, 111
Happy Birthday exercise, 97
Hawthorn, 198
Headaches, 187–89, 230

Heartbeat, fetal, 46, 211
Heartburn. *See* Indigestion
Heart palpitations, 158,
    159, 184
Hemodilution, 159
Hemoglobin, 159
Hemorrhaging, 165, 218
Hemorrhoids, 248–52
Hepatitis, 45
Herbs
  to avoid, 78, 83–85
  Chinese, 85
  common and Latin names for,
    82, 263–65
  dosages of, 83
  gathering, 82, 253–54
  for late pregnancy, 121–22
  nervine, 189
  preparing, 254–62
  purchasing, 82, 254–55, 263
  safety of, 76–77, 86
  using, during pregnancy, 77–79
  *See also individual herbs*
Herpes, 189–94
High blood pressure,
    194–98, 230
HIV, 45
Home births
  attendants at, 34–35
  history of, 4, 8
  percentage choosing, 4
  right to, 35
Hops, 221
Horse-chestnut seed extract,
    251, 252
Hospitals, births at, 34, 35
Hunger
  insomnia and, 204, 227
  paying attention to, 14, 54, 74
Hydroquinone, 235
Hyperemesis gravidarum,
    199–200
Hypertension. *See* High blood
    pressure
Hypoglycemia (low blood sugar),
    72, 180, 187, 188, 227

## I

Illnesses
  minor, 171–75
  severe, 171
  *See also individual symptoms
    and ailments*

Incontinence, 96, 233–34
Indigestion, 183, 201–3
Infusions, 256–57
Insights, creative, 30–31
Insomnia, 204–6
Insulin, 186
Intuition, 17–19, 74
Iodine, 67–68
Ipecac, 84
Irish moss, 68
Iron, 66–67
  deficiency anemia, 158–62
  headaches and, 187, 188
  Iron Tonic Syrup, 185
  sources of, 160
  supplements, 160, 161, 175
Irritability, 159, 177, 182,
    183, 184
Itchiness, 111, 207–8

## J

Joints
  frozen and stiff, 164
  looser, 112
Journal, keeping, 30, 181
Juniper berries, 84

## K

Kapha, 203
Kegel exercises, 96–97, 233
Kelp, 62, 66, 67, 68, 160
Ketones, 59
Kidney infections, 234
Kitzinger, Sheila, 8, 97
Koehler, Nan, 8
Kudzu
  for colds and flu, 174
  Garlic-Onion-Ginger-Kudzu
    Tea, 175

## L

Labor
  contractions, 183
  facilitating, 122
Lamb's quarters, 61, 156
Lang, Raven, 8
Lanugo, 22
Late pregnancy
  bleeding during, 168
  emotional changes in, 117–18
  herbs for, 121–22
  nutrition during, 121
  physical activity during, 123
  rest during, 120–21